DR. KENNETH H. COOPER

ADVANCED NUTRITIONAL THERAPIES

THOMAS NELSON PUBLISHERS
Nashville • Atlanta • London • Vancouver

Published in Nashville, Tennessee, by Thomas Nelson, Inc., Publishers, and distributed in Canada by Word Communications, Ltd., Richmond, British Columbia.

The Bible version used in this publication is THE NEW KING JAMES VERSION. Copyright © 1979, 1980, 1982, Thomas Nelson, Inc., Publishers.

Library of Congress Cataloging-in-Publication Data
Cooper, Kenneth H.
    Advanced nutritional therapies / Kenneth H. Cooper.
        p.   cm.
    Includes bibliographical references.
    ISBN 0-7852-7302-6
    1. Diet therapy—Popular works. 2. Dietary supplements—Popular works.
3. Nutrition—Popular works. I. Title.
RM216.C683   1997
615.8'54—dc21   96–45086
                                                                                       CIP

Printed in the United States of America.
1 2 3 4 5 6 — 01 00 99 98 97 96

CONTENTS

Contents

Contents

Contents

ACKNOWLEDGMENTS

The successful completion of this book required the help of a host of people, many of whom have been on my book-writing "team" in the past.

For more than fifteen years, William Proctor has served as my professional literary collaborator. Bill's abilities to organize difficult subject matter, conduct research, and prepare a finished manuscript have been essential to the last seven books I have authored. Now with this, our eighth book project together, I continue to be extremely grateful.

For nearly thirty years, my friend, agent, and editorial adviser, Herbert M. Katz, has played a decisive role in the conceptualization and preparation of all twelve of my books. His editorial creativity and sound business ability are always major factors in ushering these writing projects to a satisfying conclusion.

My heartfelt thanks also go to Nancy Katz, Herb's business partner and wife, who has played an increasingly important role in recent years in my book endeavors. In particular, Nancy has done a magnificent job of finding publishers around the world who are interested in my works, and spreading abroad the good word about the tremendous benefits of preventive medicine.

Bruce Nygren, my editor at Thomas Nelson, has again made his mark on my literary efforts. Without a steady, professional editorial hand to guide and shape the final presentation of a manuscript, the end product will almost always fall short. Bruce has edited my two previous books, *Antioxidant Revolution* and *It's Better to Believe*, and I look forward, beyond *Advanced Nutritional Therapies*, to the opportunity to work with him on other projects.

Kathryn Miller, one of our most competent dietitians at the Cooper Clinic, has again provided invaluable assistance in critiquing and editing the nutritional topics in this book. She was assisted by several of our dietetic interns, including Stacy Opitz, Lilly Pappachen, and Pam Wilson, who conducted an extensive review of the current scientific literature.

On the home front, my longtime assistant, Harriet Guthrie, has once again done an admirable job of overseeing and managing my research materials. Most important of all, she has orchestrated my busy schedule so that I could pursue still another book, despite my responsibilities with patient care, the Cooper Clinic, the Cooper Institute for Aerobics Research, and speaking engagements around the world.

Above all, I know how fortunate I am to have an understanding wife, Millie, and supportive children, Berkley and Tyler. Millie is my most trusted adviser on all matters, personal as well as business. Berkley is constantly a cheerful, upbeat source of inspiration to Dad, even as she pursues her own career and family life. As for Tyler, it's been especially satisfying to have him come on staff recently and begin to contribute in significant ways to the cause of preventive medicine.

There are many others, too numerous to name—both at the Cooper Clinic and at Thomas Nelson—who have helped with this book. I want to thank them as a group and say, on their behalf, that I trust our joint effort has produced a guide to "nutrimedicine" that will be helpful and healthful to you, my reader, and to your family and friends.

Dedication

To the many scientists and physicians who, in their laboratories, clinics, and treatment rooms, are pushing back the frontiers of our knowledge about antioxidants, and who are waging an increasingly successful war against free radicals.

PART I

THE MOST POWERFUL NUTRITIONAL THERAPIES— AND HOW THEY CAN SAVE YOUR LIFE AND HEALTH

Chapter 1

How Advanced Nutritional Therapies Can Improve Your Health, Prevent Disease, and Heal Your Body and Mind

Since ancient times, certain herbs, minerals, and other nutrients have been cloaked in mystery, revered religiously, or, in some cases, anointed with near-supernatural status because of their tremendous healing and health-giving potential. Through the trial-and-error processes of folk medicine, they have been *proven* to work on the sick, the weak, and the disturbed.

Until relatively recently, the manipulation and release of these nutritional forces resided mainly in the hands of pretechnological health practitioners, including the shaman, the medicine man, and the quasi-medical freelancer. Now, all that is changing. Scientifically trained nutrition experts and dietitians have taken us to the edge of a great medical frontier: the dynamic new world of nutrimedicine.

Even physicians, who have often been reluctant to hop

on the nutritional therapy bandwagon, now are acknowledging in ever-growing numbers that, yes, there really may be something to this nutrition business. Indeed, they concede that supplements and specific food strategies may actually prevent or overcome various diseases. Among the competing priorities that make up a successful preventive medicine program, good nutrition may now be the first among equals.

THE NEGLECTED SKILL OF "EATING SMART"

I want to invite you to join me in hands-on exploration of this exciting new field of nutritional therapy. By the time you finish this book, you may be ready to make a long-term personal commitment to learn all there is to know about the art of "eating smart," and then to apply these skills daily in your own preventive medicine program.

In fact, you may find yourself focusing on your eating habits before you consider anything else. It's certainly true that not smoking can save your life in more ways than one. It's also true that frequent exercise, regular medical checkups, stress management, and other healthy habits can contribute to a longer and better life. Yet, the neglected skill of eating intelligently is the cornerstone upon which all other healthful practices rest.

Unfortunately, few people have mastered this skill. Many people I know just eat what is put before them without thinking, and certainly without making much effort to select specific foods or distinguish food preparation styles. Even physicians are just beginning to learn how to use food to treat and protect their patients.

Using nutrition wisely requires knowledge and training. Food must be used prescriptively, as a kind of elixir that has the power to enhance energy, prevent disease, and heal the body and mind. That is why I used the term *nutrimedicine* to describe not only specific medicinal applications of certain foods and supplements, but also every meal I eat. It's also why I like to refer to the individual eating plans of my patients not simply as "meal plans," but as "nutritional therapies."

WHAT'S DIFFERENT ABOUT THIS BOOK?

This book has been designed along different lines from most other nutritional guides now on the market. When possible, I have provided scientific support and references, so that you can go to the original studies. My goal is to put your safety first by resting my case on solid research. Certainly, I have no interest in endorsing special foods, supplements, or other nutrients.

When I read a book on nutrition or preventive medicine that makes recommendations without any reference to the scientific underpinnings for the advice, I become quite uncomfortable. For this reason, you will find that I often refrain from recommending a particular item because of a lack of scientific information. I may not yet be convinced that we have enough facts to make an intelligent decision about long-term benefits and side effects.

However, I am very willing to "push the envelope" in making certain recommendations, when I think the current weight of evidence warrants my stepping out ahead of the crowd. That is the approach I have taken throughout my career. For example:

- I advocated endurance exercise and treadmill stress testing before they were popular.
- I pushed for a war on high blood cholesterol before many physicians were even doing complete blood tests on their patients.
- More recently, I have recommended the use of

antioxidants to fight the destructive effects of free radicals—the unstable oxygen molecules that may cause cancer, heart disease, and many other health problems in our bodies. For this last position, I have come under attack in some quarters of the medical community on the grounds that I have supposedly jumped the gun before all the facts are in.

My approach to preventive medicine can be summed up in a series of questions I always ask before making recommendations in this book or elsewhere:

Question 1: Is the scientific support solid for a particular recommendation I plan to make?

The operative word here is *solid*. The final word was not in on using cholesterol-lowering drugs before they began to be prescribed. Yet, many patients at risk for atherosclerosis and heart disease will be forever grateful that their cholesterol was controlled at an early stage. I am convinced there will be a similar response among those relying on antioxidant therapy and other nutritional strategies, which may not be nailed down in the scientific community.

Question 2: Is it more probable than not that consuming a certain nutrient in particular doses will provide significant health benefits?

I do not look for an airtight case that taking a particular vitamin or mineral will *definitely* result in a lowered risk of some disease. But, I do need some solid indication of a *strong likelihood* that there will be a health benefit. In the final analysis, I tend to be satisfied if most of the evidence points toward a significant and positive result.

Question 3: What, if any, are the side effects?

If the research into a certain nutrient has advanced beyond the preliminary stage but no side effects have appeared, that is usually a green light for me to give a positive recommendation. If there are side effects only at very high doses, well beyond what I suggest using, I also tend to feel comfortable giving my patients the go-ahead. But if even a small percentage of people experience problems with low doses, I will probably recommend that the nutrient not be used, or be used only under the strict supervision of a qualified physician.

Question 4: How may a particular food or supplement interact with another food, supplement, or drug?

Throughout this book, I'll be indicating how some nutrients may interact, for better or worse, with others. For example, many people should take vitamin B_{12} with folic acid supplements to prevent the possibility of pernicious anemia. (See Chapter 3 for details.) But those on a blood-thinning medication like Coumadin may want to avoid supplements that have a blood-thinning effect, such as aspirin or vitamin E. Or, they should take these supplements and medications only under the close supervision of a qualified physician.

Because I can't include every possible nutritional interaction in these pages, and you would probably find it impossible to keep track of them all if I could, be sure to inform your doctor about every supplement or special dietary strategy you are employing. This way, you can receive highly personalized advice about possible interactions.

MY PERSONAL ADVENTURES IN THE WORLD OF NUTRITION

My own systematic approach to nutritional therapy did not develop overnight. In fact, to understand how I have arrived at my position, it's necessary to take a brief excursion with me into the past, beginning with my days in medical school.

Like most physicians, I am something of a Johnny-come-lately to the nutrimedicine scene. I was never offered a course in nutrition in medical school. After I graduated from the University of Oklahoma Medical School and later the Harvard School of Public Health, I encouraged my patients to prevent disease by leading active, exercise-oriented lives, and to go in for regular medical checkups. Nutrition was only an afterthought.

Yet, within the last fifteen years, I have come to understand that every time I sit down at the dinner table, stop by our Center cafeteria, or go into the kitchen for a snack, I will either help or hurt my body. Because there is no neutral zone for food choices, it is incumbent upon me and my patients to learn what impact any given food, supplement, or other nutrient is likely to have.

My deep conviction about nutrition is not the result of a dramatic, one-time epiphany. Rather, my sensitivities in this area have emerged gradually over a period of years. The culmination of my personal transformation was my best-seller, *Controlling Cholesterol* (Bantam, 1988), which focused in large part on the destructive, heart-endangering role of saturated fats and high-cholesterol foods in the diet.

A little later, while authoring *Preventing Osteoporosis* (Bantam, 1989), I was impressed, as are many other preventive medicine specialists, by the central role of calcium, including calcium supplements, in protecting us from the bone-thinning disease that afflicts an estimated 24 million Americans. But I quickly became aware that total calcium intake was only part of the story. For one thing, I was struck how the effectiveness of calcium can be multiplied by combining it with exercise or hormone replacement therapy. This synergistic interaction of food with other factors is a theme that emerges again and again in this book.

My adventures in the world of nutrition continued with *Overcoming Hypertension* (Bantam, 1991). There, with Dr. Norman Kaplan, world-famous expert on high blood pressure, I examined an array of foods and nutrients including sodium, potassium, calcium, fats, and even licorice, which can influence blood pressure. In *Advanced Nutritional Therapies*, I have updated many of those insights. More recently, my *Antioxidant Revolution* (Nelson, 1994) explored the ways that vitamins E, C, beta-carotene, and other antioxidants can be used to fight free radicals—those unstable oxygen molecules that constantly bombard our tissues, blood vessels, and even our cells and genetic codes. As they arise in the body and inflict damage through pollution, stress, excessive exercise and traumatic injuries, free radicals threaten us with cancers, heart disease, immune disorders, and other potentially lethal illnesses. A wise application of nutritional therapy can provide an effective front line of defense.

As a result of my growing belief in the power of nutrition, I am acutely aware of the importance of every mouthful of food I take. For example, I know that the five to seven servings of fruits and vegetables I have every day are packed with the vitamins, minerals, and other nutrients I need to support my exercise and other energy needs. I also know that if I have one cup of commercial vegetable soup for lunch, I will certainly take in plenty of antioxidants and other important nutrients, but I will also use up about one-fourth of my sodium limit for the day. Finally, I know that by eating that extra piece of steak or a fat-filled dessert, I will, even if ever so slightly, raise my risk of colon cancer, heart disease, and other problems.

BEYOND THE ANTIOXIDANT REVOLUTION

To be sure, such goals as controlling cholesterol, limiting saturated fats, keeping calcium intake high, reducing salt for those who are "salt-sensitive," and emphasizing a diet high in antioxidants continue to be primary concerns for me. But this book goes several steps beyond these goals.

Much has happened in the world of nutrition research in the short time since *Antioxidant Revolution* was published. For one thing, there is mounting evidence that excessive exercise without the protection of antioxidants can put you at risk for many life-threatening diseases. In addition, the antioxidant vitamin E has assumed even greater importance for its power to protect against heart disease. On the other hand, questions have been raised about beta-carotene and even about high doses of vitamin C. (For my evaluations and recommendations, see Chapter 4.)

The many new nutritional issues make it imperative for me to publish this book. Here is a sampling:

- Folic acid (folate), a member of the B vitamin complex, may be on the verge of taking center stage in the fight against heart disease.

Among other things, folate lowers the blood levels of homocysteines, amino acids that have been implicated in the buildup of plaque in the vessels. Also, folic acid has been linked to protection against birth defects, stroke, kidney disease, cancer, degeneration of the spinal cord, and many other serious health conditions. (For more, see Chapters 2 and 3.)

- Melatonin, a hormonal secretion of the pineal gland in the brain, has emerged as a popular but highly controversial supplement.

Identified by some researchers as a powerful antioxidant, melatonin has been used successfully as a treatment for insomnia and jet lag. But its staunchest advocates have also touted it for other curative possibilities, including cancer treatment, overcoming immune disorders, and even retarding the aging process. (For more information, see the "Melatonin" entry in Chapter 6.)

- Phytoestrogens, the plant-based hormones that are transformed into mild estrogens in the body, can significantly relieve the hot flushes of menopause and other complaints. But are they safe? (See the "Hormones" entry in Chapter 6.)

Some of these topics are discussed in more detail in the remainder of Part I. As you move on to Part II, you will find an alphabetized guide to nutritional therapy, providing easy-to-apply suggestions for using different foods, supplements, and nutrients to treat health problems and achieve protection from various diseases.

Nutrimedicine is such a new medical discipline that it doesn't even exist as a separate specialty, but neither did preventive medicine when I set up the first treadmill in Dallas, or when I began to advocate aerobic exercise as an essential component of a strong, personal preventive medicine program. Now, preventive medicine *is* a recognized medical specialty.

I believe it will only be a matter of time before the nutritional therapies introduced in this book become an established part of medical practice. In the meantime, follow these guidelines to protect yourself:

- Avoid unsubstantiated claims, and demand scientific authority for every recommendation you hear or read.
- Ascertain that any new nutritional therapy is supported by solid research.
- Beware of possible side effects, and undergo regular medical exams and blood tests from your physician.
- Whenever possible, learn how foods and supplements interact with one another or with other drugs.
- Above all, you must learn to rely on what is *known* about nutrition—what has been proven to some extent and has the backing of reputable physicians

and registered dietitians. The last word doesn't have to be in on a particular vitamin, mineral, or food item before you decide to use it. But when you are taking advantage of groundbreaking research, you must discipline yourself to stay alert, be discerning, and always check any questionable advice with your doctor. With this approach, you will be in a position to make wise decisions about your health as you take advantage of the latest developments in nutrition.

Keep in mind that half of all deaths in the United States are the result of an unhealthy lifestyle, which we, individually and as a society, can change. This means that all of us must assume more responsibility for our own health and not rely only on a physician or the government. Rather, to manage our health more effectively and to make better informed decisions, we need up-to-date and accurate information—and that is exactly what I am trying to provide for you in this book.

Chapter 2

The Folic Acid Factor

The most promising new player on the nutritional scene right now is folic acid, a member of the B-complex vitamin family, which is produced primarily by plants and yeast.

Also called "folate," a deficiency of this nutrient has been linked in recent scientific studies to a wide variety of diseases and health conditions, including:

- Neural-tube birth defects such as spina bifida and anencephaly
- Congenital abnormalities, including cleft palate and heart and limb defects
- Atherosclerosis or clogging of the arteries
- Heart attacks
- Stroke
- Kidney disorders
- Cervical dysplasia (abnormal tissue development) and possibly cervical cancer

The main way that folate protects you is by lowering the levels of "homocysteines" in your blood. These are amino acids that have been associated with damage to cells lining the vessel walls.

To reduce the risk of homocysteines, the evidence suggests that everyone should take at least 400 *micro*grams of folate per day. (One milligram equals 1,000 micrograms; so 400 micrograms equals 0.4 milligrams.) People in high-risk categories for certain diseases or health problems, those who have already had a child with a neural-tube defect, or who have exceptionally high levels of homocysteines, should take considerably more folate.

The minimum amount of folate can easily be obtained by making certain adjustments to the average diet. For example, one cup of wheat flakes cereal contains more than 400 micrograms of folic acid; one cup of cooked baby lima beans provides 273 micrograms; one cup of cranberries has 366 micrograms; and one cup of cooked black-eyed peas has 209 micrograms.

As you can see, paying just a little more attention to your daily food intake will probably allow you to go beyond the minimum intake of folate every day. But for those who have trouble getting a full 400 micrograms through meals, or who need higher doses because of higher health risks, folic acid is also available through small, inexpensive tablets sold over the counter in most pharmacies or supermarkets.

What is the evidence for folate? As I mentioned in Chapter 1, I don't expect you to rely wholly on my opinion about folate or anything else. I make a recommendation only when I feel the weight of the scientific research warrants such a recommendation. So now, let's take a look at how solid the scientific support is for this B-complex powerhouse.

WHAT'S THE SCIENTIFIC EVIDENCE FOR FOLATE?

An adequate intake of folic acid is absolutely necessary for *everyone*, male or female. But the first significant wave of research involving this vitamin focused on women, and particularly women of childbearing age.

The Female Factor

An estimated 4,000 children, born and unborn, are diagnosed annually in the United States with neural-tube defects. These include spina bifida (a malformation and lack of fusion of the spinal canal) and anencephaly (a condition where the child is born without a brain).

Yet these tragedies are not inevitable. Prospective mothers who increase their intake of folic acid could prevent one-half to three-quarters of these sad cases, according to an editorial in the *Journal of the American Medical Association* (December 6, 1995, p. 1717).

In the 1960s, researchers suspected that folate played a critical role in preventing neural-tube defects and other birth abnormalities. But it wasn't until 1992 that the U.S. Public Health Service recommended that *all* women who might become pregnant take a daily dose of 400 micrograms of folate. Unfortunately, only 15 percent of these women who are at risk know about this recommendation, according to a 1995 March of Dimes study.

A related problem is that at the present time, the official Recommended Dietary Allowance (RDA) for folate lags behind the above recommendation from the Public Health Service. Specifically, the RDA remains at 400 mcg daily for pregnant women, 180 mcg for nonpregnant adult women, and 260 to 280 mcg for women who are lactating (nursing their babies). Also, the folate RDA for adult men is 200 mcg daily.

In fact, many women take in much less than the required minimum amount of folate—less than 300 micrograms per day by some estimates. As a result, various studies have shown that 15 to 30 percent of young women have blood levels of folic acid that are too low.

For women who have already had a pregnancy involving a child with a neural-tube defect and are planning another pregnancy, it's important to rely even more heavily on folate to prevent a recurrence of the problem. National medical committees now recommend supplements of 4 to 5 *milli*grams (4,000-5,000 micrograms) per day for these women before conception and during the early months of pregnancy. (See *Journal of the American Medical Association,* December 6, 1995, pp. 1698-1702.)

Caution: Although folic acid has no known direct side effects, it should only be given in therapeutic doses greater than 400 micrograms daily after pernicious anemia has been ruled out. The only exceptions to this rule are for pregnant and lactating (nursing) women, who may be taking large doses under the care of a physician.

The reason for this rule is that patients with pernicious anemia who are taking more than 400 micrograms of folic acid daily may develop severe and possibly irreversible neurological abnormalities if they are inadequately treated with vitamin B_{12}. Adequate doses of B_{12}, which usually must be taken by injection since very large oral supplements are required, may prevent, halt, or improve the neurological changes caused by pernicious anemia. (See Chapter 3 for my specific recommendations.)

The Heart of the Matter

Folic acid is not just for childbearing females and their offspring. A broader benefit, which applies to men and women of all ages, is more a matter of the heart. In analyzing thirty-eight studies on folic acid in a 1995 article for the *Journal of the American Medical Association,* a research group from the University of Washington found that taking folic acid can reduce the levels of the amino acid homocysteine in the blood. This lowering of homocysteines will, in turn, reduce the risks of heart disease, blood vessel disease, and strokes. (See *JAMA*, October 14, 1995, pp. 1049-57.)

The Washington researchers concluded that up to 50,000 artery disease deaths could be avoided each year if homocysteines were lowered through increased intake of dietary folate in such foods as yeast, brussels sprouts, asparagus, and soybean sprouts. The daily dose is also available in folic acid supplements and in foods fortified with folate. In fact, the U.S. Food and Drug Administration announced in March 1996 that it will require all enriched foods to be fortified with folic acid beginning in January 1998. This will include breads, flour, cornmeal, pasta, rice, and many other grain products.

Some estimates suggest that deficiencies in folic acid may trigger 30 to 40 percent of the heart attacks and strokes suffered by men in the United States each year. A high homocysteine level, which can be corrected by folate, is an independent risk factor for coronary artery disease. In other words, your homocysteine level can, by itself, significantly raise your risk of heart disease. Homocysteine level is also an independent risk factor in identifying a tendency for the members of certain families to suffer coronary disease at a particularly early age. (See *Arteriosclerotic Thrombosis in Vascular Biology*, September 1995, pp. 1314-20.)

Many experts feel that the homocysteine levels in the blood may actually become as important as cholesterol in signaling the clogging of the arteries and heart disease! We'll go into the issue of homocysteine testing and levels in more detail in the following chapter.

What Else Can Folate Do?

A series of recent scientific studies has suggested that there are other possible health benefits from folic acid. Here are some of them:

- *Special help for the elderly:* The balance of the scientific evidence suggests that the elderly could benefit from injections of low doses of vitamin B_{12} (cobalamin) or from folate supplements, according to a 1995 report from Queens University, Kingston, Ontario, Canada. (See *Baillieres Clinical Haematology*, September 1995, pp. 679-97.) Through such treatments, older people can be protected from damage to their blood vessels from elevated homocysteines and also from damage to the nervous system from pernicious anemia.
- *Tumors:* There is mounting evidence that low folate levels may be associated with increased risks of tumor growth (neoplasia), as well as vessel disease and birth defects. (See *Baillieres Clinical Haematology*, September, 1995, pp. 533-66.)
- *Cancer:* Folate deficiency significantly increases chromosome breaks in human DNA, the genetic code of our cells. This finding by scientists at the University of New South Wales, Kensington, Australia, is consistent with other clinical and epidemiological evidence linking folate deficiency to DNA damage and cancer. (See *Baillieres Clinical Haematology*, September 1995, pp. 461-78.) A related report in the September 1995 issue of *Medical Hypotheses* (pp. 297-303) suggested that cancer can be initiated by DNA damage resulting from folic acid deficiency. According to the author, low levels of folic acid in North American diets may be a factor causing many cancers. A considerable body of research points to links between folate deficiency and cervical dysplasia—a precancerous condition of the cervix. (See *Journal of the American College of Nutrition*, Gusut, 1993, pp. 438-41.)
- *Spinal cord degeneration:* In rare cases, a folate

deficiency may result in degeneration of the spinal cord. In a case followed by researchers at the Meridia Huron Hospital, East Cleveland, Ohio, a thirty-nine-year-old man experienced disturbances in his walking gait, general weakness, confusion, and depression. He was also bed-bound, suffered from a loss of a sense of his body position, and felt vibrations in his lower extremities. As it happened, for more than two years he had been taking phenobarbital, a sleep-inducing barbiturate that can cause folate deficiency. So for four months, his physicians treated him with folate and intravenous injections of red blood cells (erythrocytes). The result was overall improvement, with a return of his ability to walk, a normal sense of position, and virtual elimination of the vibration in his legs. (See *American Journal of Medical Science*, November 1995, pp. 214-6.)

- *Failure to recover from surgery:* An obese fifty-one-year-old woman underwent surgery, but after fifty-two days in the hospital, she still suffered from a variety of problems. These included: infections, sore tongue, altered sense of taste, severe weight loss, diarrhea, poor appetite, depressed mood, and a liver abscess. Her doctors discovered that she had a folate deficiency, and that her regular diet was chronically low in folate. Also, she had been undergoing estrogen therapy for fifteen years—treatment that may deplete the body of folate. The physicians began to give her vitamin and mineral supplements, including folic acid. Within a month, her nutritional status and overall health improved dramatically. The doctors concluded that her poor diet, long-term estrogen use, stress from surgery, and lingering infections may have contributed to her folate deficiency and her prolonged hospital stay. (See *Nutrition and Clinical Practice*, December 1994, pp. 247-50.)

- *Kidney disease:* Scientists at the Department of Internal Medicine, Krankenhous der Barmherzigen Bruder, Eisenstadt, Austria, reported in 1995 that the administration of folic acid to patients with chronic renal (kidney) disease will enhance the effectiveness of their therapy. In this particular case, folate enabled the other drug dosages to be reduced. (See *Nephron*, 1995, pp. 395-400.)
- *Heart and limb birth defects:* A 1995 March of Dimes study found that women who take multivitamins with folic acid and who eat fortified cereals at the time of their conception have a 30 to 35 percent lower risk of delivering offspring with heart defects or limb defects. (See *American Journal of Medicine and Genetics*, December 4, 1995, pp. 536-45.)

A GUIDE TO THE BEST SOURCES OF FOLATE

There are two ways to obtain folic acid, or any other vitamin or mineral, for that matter: through the food you eat or through a supplement.

Whenever possible, always choose the food route. Despite the advances in nutrition research, there is still a great deal that we don't know about the impact of separating a particular nutrient from its food context. I believe that other nutrients in food support and enhance the action of folate.

We do have evidence that folate tablets can have a beneficial effect on health. As you will see in the next chapter, I recommend that everyone take at least 400 micrograms of folate per day in the form of supplements. There is simply no point in taking any chance on failing to get the minimum amount into your system.

Still, even if you take supplements, I strongly recommend that you also adjust your diet so that it is high in folic acid. I've already mentioned a number of foods that are high in folate, but here is a more complete list, with approximate amounts of the vitamin in micrograms per serving:

Beans:
    Cranberry beans, one cup (boiled)-366 mcg
    Black-eyed peas, one cup (cooked)-209 mcg
    Pinto beans, one cup-292 mcg
    Garbanzo beans (chickpeas), one cup (cooked)-
       282 mcg
    Baby lima beans, one cup (cooked)-273 mcg
    Black beans, one cup (cooked)-256 mcg
    Navy beans, one cup (cooked)-255 mcg
    Small white beans, one cup (cooked)-246 mcg
    Kidney beans, one cup (cooked)-229 mcg
    Great Northern beans, one cup (cooked)-180 mcg
    Large lima beans, one cup (cooked)-156 mcg

Cereals:
    Fortified bran flakes, one cup (dry)-133 mcg
    Corn flakes, one cup (dry)-100 mcg
    Fortified oat flakes, one cup (dry)-133 mcg
    Wheat flakes cereal, one cup (dry)-400 mcg
    Toasted wheat germ, one cup (dry)-300 mcg

Other foods:
    Soybean flour (defatted), one cup-305 mcg
    Avocado (California), one-113 mcg
    Orange, one-40 mcg
    Cantaloupe, one-half-45 mcg
    Pineapple juice, one cup-60 mcg
    Beef liver, 4 ounces (cooked)-248 mcg
    Chicken liver, one (cooked)-220 mcg
    Lentil soup with ham (cooked), 2 ounces-50 mcg
    Asparagus, one cup (cooked)-90 mcg

Beets, one cup (cooked)-90 mcg
Broccoli, one cup (cooked)-98 mcg
Brussels sprouts, one cup (cooked)-94 mcg
Cauliflower, one cup (cooked)-65 mcg
Corn, one cup (cooked)-70 mcg
Okra, one cup (cooked)-74 mcg
Soybean sprouts, one cup (cooked)-193 mcg
Brewer's yeast, 1 tablespoon-313 mcg
Turnip greens, one cup-110 mcg

By this time, you have a good idea about what folic acid can do, and you know some of the best food sources that should be a part of your diet. But considerably more needs to be said about homocysteines—how to test for them, what your blood ranges should be, and exactly how much folate and vitamin B_{12} you should be taking into your system every day.

Chapter 3

The Homocysteine Checkup— and a Guide to Folate Therapy

Nobody's talking about it, your doctor hasn't heard of it, but there is something in your blood that could be even more dangerous than cholesterol. This time, however, the cure is simple."

These provocative words from *Health* (September 1995, p. 69) may sound so sensational or even unrealistic that you might question whether they should be included in a reputable health publication. But they happen to be accurate.

The topic being referred to is *homocysteine*, a word that hasn't yet entered the vocabulary of most people, including many physicians. In the near future, however, it is virtually certain that most physicians will do routine checks on homocysteine levels for those patients at high risk for atherosclerosis or heart disease.

As you know from the previous chapter, homocysteine is a sulphur-containing amino acid that has been linked to several medical problems, including severe damage to the walls of blood vessels and diseases like artery-clogging atherosclerosis (also commonly called "arteriosclerosis"). The scientific evidence against homocysteine has been steadily mounting in major articles, which began appearing in the medical literature in early 1995.

THE LATEST INDICTMENTS OF HOMOCYSTEINE

Here is a sampling of what the scientists are saying about this threatening amino acid: One 1995 study clearly showed a relationship between high blood levels of homocysteine and obstructions in the carotid arteries, which are the vessels in the neck supplying blood to the brain. (See the *New England Journal of Medicine*, February 2, 1995, pp. 286-9.)

Another report demonstrated an excellent correlation between blood levels of homocysteine and generalized arteriosclerosis, or hardening of the arteries. Furthermore, the researchers determined that even moderate levels of folic acid could rapidly lower the homocysteine levels. They said that reducing homocysteine levels by increasing the intake of folic acid "promises to prevent arteriosclerotic vascular disease." (*Journal of the American Medical Association*, October 4, 1995, pp. 1049-57.)

Still another study, published in late 1995, showed a relationship among cigarette smoking, elevated cholesterol, high blood pressure, inactivity, and high homocysteine levels. (*JAMA*, November 15, 1995, p. 15.) But even if there is a link that ties these factors together, researchers are also concluding that the effect of homocysteine is so powerful that it can operate independently of such risk factors as high cholesterol or hypertension.

Specifically, a high homocysteine level may reflect inadequate availability in the human body of any one of three important vitamins—folic acid, vitamin B_6, or vitamin

B_{12}. Supplementation with these vitamins, particularly folic acid, can lower homocysteine levels to normal. But further studies are needed to establish for certain that lowering high homocysteine levels will definitely lead to a reduction in cardiovascular risk.

Scientific studies have also established a relationship between blood levels of folate and fatal coronary heart disease. A report published on June 26, 1996, in the *Journal of the American Medical Association* (pp. 1893-6), focused on 5,056 Canadian men and women, aged 35 to 79. The researchers found a significant relationship between low serum folate levels and an increased risk of fatal coronary heart disease.

These and other studies are making it clear that an important new frontier has been identified in the ongoing fight against heart disease. But I know from personal experience, including my early encounters with cholesterol and other serious challenges to our health, that it takes time for the weight of the evidence to be felt throughout the practicing medical community.

From Controlling Cholesterol to Harnessing Homocysteines

In the mid to late seventies, a few medical centers, including our Cooper Clinic in Dallas, would test for total cholesterol levels. But in those days, no one really knew what degree of risk should be associated with given levels of cholesterol. Also, little was known about the importance of the subcomponents of total cholesterol such as the "good" HDL (high-density lipoprotein) cholesterol, and the "bad" LDL (low-density lipoprotein) cholesterol.

For a long time, most physicians just assumed that as long as your cholesterol wasn't higher than 250 to 300 milligrams per deciliter, you were probably in the safe range. It wasn't until well into the 1980s that the safe threshold of

200 mg/dl was established. Also, at about that time we became more aware of the importance of the ratio of total cholesterol to HDL cholesterol as a predictor of vessel disease risk. (See my *Controlling Cholesterol* for more detailed information on this issue.)

In many ways, public knowledge of the danger of homocysteine and how to harness and control it is at the early stage that characterized our understanding of cholesterol in the late 1970s and early 1980s. But despite the research and clinical observation that still needs to be done, we know enough now to reveal the "homocysteine secret," and to make some recommendations about harnessing the potentially destructive action of this amino acid.

Revealing the Homocysteine Secret

Inside your body, an incredible, tumultuous, three-ring circus is taking place. Various chemicals, enzymes, amino acids (the "building blocks" of protein), unstable oxygen molecules known as "free radicals," and electrical charges are constantly bouncing back and forth. At blinding speed, they crash into one another, combining and creating, causing life to move forward—or backward. The action is so explosive and wide-ranging that it's impossible to keep track of everything that is occurring, even with the most sophisticated instruments now available to scientists.

Despite all the seemingly chaotic and confusing activity, when everything is working properly on the molecular level in our bodies, a delicate balance is achieved. There is just the right number of amino acids, just the right amount of action-triggering chemicals and enzymes, and just the right quantity of chemical by-products that can be safely washed out of our systems.

Unfortunately, things are not always in perfect balance. The problem may be the genetic code we inherited from our parents or other ancestors. We may have acquired a tendency to have too much of one type of chemical, or perhaps a deficiency in the way our bodies process, metabolize, or use an amino acid or enzyme.

Also, chemical malfunctions and imbalances may occur as we grow older, consume a poor diet, or are exposed to pollution, sunlight, stress, or excessive exercise. Such factors can cause the molecular performers inside us to misbehave. To carry the circus image a step further, the "star performers" begin to operate outside the "rings" to which they were assigned, and serious diseases and death may be the final result.

Like cholesterol, homocysteine is one of the important molecular players inside our bodies. As such, it is not inherently bad. In fact, as one of the all-important amino acids, or building blocks of protein, homocysteine appears in the body as a necessary by-product of the breakdown of the "essential" amino acid methionine. (An essential amino acid is one that cannot be produced by the body, but must be brought in from the outside, through food or supplements.)

Furthermore, homocysteine engages in chemical interactions involving methionine and another amino acid, cysteine. In this role, homocysteine operates as a kind of transition player, contributing to the step-by-step biosynthesis (or formation of chemical compounds by enzymes) of cysteine from methionine.

But once again, somewhat like cholesterol, homocysteine may lose its balance because of inherited flaws, poor diet, or any of the reasons suggested above. According to the latest research, the main threat we face is *too much* homocysteine.

What Happens If You Have Too Much Homocysteine?

Evidence has accumulated to the point of near certainty that elevated blood levels of homocysteine increase the risk of atherosclerosis, a clogging of the arteries that is the major factor in the majority of heart attacks and strokes. In fact, elevated homocysteine levels are found in 25 percent of heart attack patients and 40 percent of stroke victims.

The original hypothesis for this idea was proposed by K. S. McCully in the *American Journal of Pathology* in 1969. He suggested the causal link after doing postmortem studies on a group of people with high homocysteine levels who also suffered from atherosclerosis (or clogging of the arteries). The medical establishment has now placed its stamp of approval on this position. A recent editorial in the prestigious *New England Journal of Medicine* (February 2, 1995, pp. 328-29), citing many studies published since McCully's report, generally accepted the cause-and-effect relationship between homocysteine and atherosclerosis.

Several possible mechanisms have been suggested for how too much homocysteine can cause vessel disease:

- Homocysteine may cause direct damage through a toxic effect on the lining of the blood vessels. In other words, it rips and tears away at them, leaving them open to the accumulation of plaque and clogging.
- Homocysteine may stimulate the development of a "smooth-muscle cell," a key component in the onset of atherosclerosis.
- Homocysteine may act as a "thrombogenic agent," triggering blood clots that can block the arteries.
- Excess homocysteine may release free radicals, which proceed to damage the vessel walls and pave the way for atherosclerosis. (See a Swedish study in *Biochim-Biophys Acta*, October 19, 1995, pp. 6-12.)
- Homocysteine may promote the oxidation of "bad" LDL cholesterol through iron in the blood, and then encourage the development of premature

atherosclerosis. (See *Free Radical Research*, October 1994, pp. 267-76.)
- High homocysteine levels may promote the presence of too much "bad" LDL cholesterol in the blood. The LDL is then "gobbled up" by white blood cells (macrophages), and the LDL-gorged white blood cells are deposited as plaque on the vessel walls. (See *Annals of Clinical Laboratories of Science*, November-December 1993, pp. 477-93.)

Whatever the precise mechanism, out-of-control homocysteine poses a serious threat to your circulatory system.

, Furthermore, too much homocysteine may be the main problem in neural-tube defects. Since the early 1980s, evidence has been building that a lack of folate in the blood contributes to birth problems like spina bifida. (See *Journal of the American Medical Association*, December 6, 1995, pp. 1698-1702, and also the discussion in the previous chapter.)

Scientists are still searching for the precise mechanism that produces these defects. But more and more, suspicion is being cast on amino acid interactions involving methionine and homocysteine. One idea is that an enzyme, methionine synthase, is the culprit. Another candidate is homocysteine itself. Here are a couple of possibilities:

- The ability of homocysteine to interact with methionine may become impaired at a crucial stage of fetal growth. (See *Nutritional Review*, June 1995, pp. 173-5.)
- A 1995 Dutch study concluded that the cause of neural-tube defects in newborns could be a defect in the mother's or child's homocysteine metabolism. (See *American Journal of Obstetrics and Gynecology*, May 1995, pp. 1436-41.)

A breakdown in the homocysteine mechanism has also been associated with problems other than heart disease and birth defects. For example, Norwegian researchers at the University of Oslo reported in a 1996 study of HIV-infected patients that elevated concentrations of homocysteine could possibly contribute to formation of "reactive oxygen species" (free radicals). The free radicals might, in turn, accelerate the deterioration of the body's immune system. (See *American Journal of Clinical Nutrition*, February 1996, pp. 242-8.)

A high concentration of homocysteine has even been associated with poor cognitive skills. In a 1996 report on an elderly group at the Research Center on Aging at Tufts University, researchers found a strong association between lower spatial copying performance and high homocysteine levels. (See *American Journal of Clinical Nutrition*, March 1996, pp. 306-14.)

Other diseases or conditions that may be linked to high homocysteine levels include:

- Advanced renal (kidney) disease. (See *Atherosclerosis*, April 7, 1995, pp. 93-103.)
- Schizophrenia. (See *Journal of Neural Transmissions and Genetics Section*, 1994, pp. 143-52.)
- Cancer. (See *Annals of Clinical Laboratories of Science*, March-April 1994, pp. 134-52.)
- Aging. (See *Journal of the American Medical Association*, December 8, 1993, pp. 2693-8.)
- Spontaneous abortions and early pregnancy loss. (See *Fertilization and Sterilization*, November 1993, pp. 820-5.)

These, then, are some of the ways that high homocysteine levels can wreak havoc in your body. But what exactly is "high" and what is "low"? Although scientists are still studying the meaning of different measurements of this amino acid in human plasma, enough is now known for you to be able to evaluate your status.

Measuring Your Homocysteines

Most physicians don't routinely provide their patients with homocysteine measurements. The concept is too new, and laboratory facilities that do the tests often aren't readily available. Your doctor should be able to arrange for a test, but blood samples may have to be shipped to a distant location, and it is costly. The charge for a test currently runs as high as $137.

In any case, here is what we now know about the test: Homocysteine is measured in "micromoles per liter." The "acceptable" or "normal" range reported by many laboratories generally runs from 5 micromoles per liter to about 20 micromoles per liter.

Unfortunately, this 5 to 20 "normal" value isn't so normal, according to the latest research. In fact, in the Physicians' Health Study reported in the *Journal of the American Medical Association* in 1992, those with plasma levels above 15.8 had a threefold greater risk of heart attack than those with lower levels. In most studies, experts have considered the "red" or danger zone to be 14 or higher.

Furthermore, in another study by Dr. Paul Hopkins of the University of Utah Cardiovascular Genetics Research Clinic, men with homocysteine levels of 19 or more were fourteen times more likely to have coronary artery disease than those with levels of 9 or less. (See *Internal Medicine News*, November 1, 1995, p. 7.)

A number of other studies have indicated that the lower your homocysteine level, the better. Any increase apparently tends to increase your risk of cardiovascular disease, and probably many other homocysteine-related diseases as well.

From these and other studies, I would suggest these homocysteine risk ranges for cardiovascular disease, as well as other homocysteine-related diseases:

> 5 micromoles per liter or lower—low risk
> 6-9 micromoles per liter—very low risk
> 10-12 micromoles per liter—moderate risk
> 13-18 micromoles per liter—high risk
> 19 micromoles per liter or higher—very high risk

Suppose your homocysteine levels are in the higher ranges. What can you do about it? The first answer is folate therapy.

INTRODUCTION TO FOLATE THERAPY

Now, the time has arrived to put it all together—to combine what we know about folic acid and homocysteine and come up with some practical recommendations that you can incorporate into your personal preventive medicine program.

First of all, here are some basic principles and points to keep in mind:

- I recommend the minimum amount of folic acid that *everyone* should be taking in every day is 400 micrograms. Everyone should get at least this minimum through a folic acid supplement, and at the same time, consume plenty of foods high in folate. (See the list in Chapter 2.) This way, you will be sure to take in the minimum and also benefit from extra folic acid through your diet.

Caution: This minimum is *imperative* for women of childbearing age. Neural-tube defects occur just after conception, and yet most women don't become aware they are pregnant until a few weeks after conception. So it's important for women in this category to be on folic acid constantly and not take a chance that they may begin their dosages too late.

- Women who have already had a child with a neural-tube defect should take folic acid supplements of 4 to 5 *milli*grams per day (or 4,000 to 5,000 micro-grams).

Caution: This amount of folate should be taken only under the supervision of a physician. Typically, you begin taking these large doses about four weeks before pregnancy and continue the therapy through the first three months.

In general, large doses of folic acid have no known toxic effects. Rarely, however, there may be instances of allergic responses, including erythema (red skin), skin rashes, itching, general malaise, and perhaps even respiratory difficulty due to spasms in the airway. If you have any questions about one or more of these reactions, immediately consult with a physician.

Also, any Folic acid dose above 1,000 micrograms daily can mask pernicious anemia, which develops because of a lack of the "intrinsic factor." This factor prevents vitamin B_{12} food sources from being absorbed. Consequently, regular injections of vitamin B_{12} may be necessary to treat diagnosed cases of pernicious anemia. Oral B_{12} supplements are also important in preventing pernicious anemia and in treating patients with borderline vitamin deficiencies. In any event, your daily diet should include plenty of vitamin B_{12}. (For a listing of foods that are rich in this vitamin see the entry under this topic in Part II.)

Symptoms of pernicious anemia include inflammation of the tip of the tongue, nervous disorders such as mood disturbances and impaired reflexes, poor memory, overall weakness, and a feeling of pins and needles in the skin. If the condition isn't corrected, permanent nerve damage may result.

Here are some additional points that have influenced my Folate therapy recommendations:

- Because pernicious anemia is more common among men and women who are fifty and older, I recommend that people in this age range who are taking folic acid also take 500 micrograms of vitamin B_{12} daily.

- The amount of vitamin B_{12} you should take is roughly 200 micrograms per day for every 1,000 micrograms of folic acid. No problems have been seen for people getting extra B_{12}, but still, for the precise dosage, see your physician.

- Vitamin B_6 (pyridoxine) deficiency has also been associated with lower levels of homocysteine in the blood. As a result, I recommend that everyone take in at least the RDA of 2.0 milligrams per day of this vitamin. The average person who is not in any special risk category can get this nutrient through supplements or through food, though B_6 may be destroyed through cooking. For foods containing this vitamin, see "Vitamin B_6" in Part II.

Caution: Megadoses of B_6 (around 100 milligrams) have caused nerve damage.

The Folate Therapy Recommendations

With this background in mind, here are my specific recommendations for daily dosages. Unless otherwise indicated, the nutrients recommended should be taken in the form of supplements. But at the same time, care should also be taken to eat plenty of foods containing the vitamins.

- Men and women under fifty with homocysteine in the low to low-moderate range: 400 micrograms of folic acid per day.

Note: This dosage is absolutely imperative for women of childbearing age.

In addition, those in this category should take in at least 200 micrograms of vitamin B_{12} and 2.0 milligrams of vitamin B_6 per day. For very low and low-risk people, these nutrients may be taken in through the diet, rather than supplements.

- Men and women of any age with homocysteine in the moderate to high range: 800-1,000 micrograms of folic acid, plus 500-1,000 micrograms of vitamin B_{12}, plus 50 milligrams of vitamin B_6 in supplement form every day.
- Men and women of any age with homocysteine values in the very high range should see a physician for treatment. Most likely, higher dosages of folic acid, and supplements of vitamins B_{12} and B_6 will be required.
- Women who have had a previous pregnancy involving a child with a neural-birth defect should take much higher doses of folic acid, in the 4,000 to 5,000 micrograms per day range—under medical supervision. Also, they should take proportionally larger amounts of vitamins B_{12} and B_6. For the specific prescription you need, see your physician. Remember, if there is a vitamin B_{12} deficiency, pernicious anemia may develop when high doses of folic acid are not offset with doses of vitamin B_{12}.
- Men and women fifty and older who do not fall into any of the high-risk categories should take 800 micrograms of folic acid, 500 micrograms of vitamin B_{12}, and 50 milligrams of vitamin B_6 per day.

As far as heart disease is concerned, having high homocysteine levels is about as dangerous as smoking. With women, homocysteines rise around the time of menopause, but there is an antidote: Estrogen-like hormones and drugs may shield women by helping rid their bodies of homocysteines. With men, as well as women, homocysteine levels continue to increase with age.

As I've already indicated, homocysteines arise from the breakdown of another amino acid, methionine, which is taken into the body through meat and dairy products. So it stands to reason that reducing the intake of meats and high-fat dairy products may help limit the body's production of homocysteine.

Although such dietary and hormonal treatments may be used to counter high homocysteine levels, the most powerful preventive response now known is folic acid. This is one of those rare occasions where we know the cure before we really understand the disease. A minimum of 13,500 deaths annually from coronary artery disease could be prevented by increasing folate intake to reduce blood homocysteine levels.

By pursuing nutritional therapy with folate and the related B vitamins, you will go a long way toward protecting yourself from heart disease, birth defects, cancer, and many other threats to your health. Furthermore, you add one more antioxidant weapon to your arsenal in your lifelong fight against free radicals.

But obviously, folic acid is only part of the antioxidant story. For the latest on advanced antioxidant therapy, turn the page.

Chapter 4

The Changing Landscape of Antioxidant Therapy

Much has happened since my *Antioxidant Revolution* was published in 1994. Now, most people actually seem to have heard about antioxidants; they associate them with vitamins E, C, and beta-carotene and know that somehow, these nutrients are able to protect their bodies from the onslaught of free radicals. These are major strides forward from the days when the usual response was a blank look when I simply mentioned the word *antioxidant!*

Still, I find that in any discussion of this topic, I have to begin by reminding my patients and readers about a few basic facts. To begin with, antioxidants are nutrients that fight off free radicals, those unstable oxygen molecules that are constantly bombarding our bodies as a result of pollution, psychological stress, excessive exercise, traumatic injuries, and a variety of other negative factors. Unless those free radicals are neutralized, our risk of suffering more than fifty diseases, including atherosclerosis, heart attacks, various cancers, and cataracts, increases considerably.

Our bodies produce a variety of antioxidants to fight free radicals, but they need help from the outside, through a well-managed diet and a supplement program. Specifically, the most powerful antioxidants we can take in through foods and supplements are vitamin E, vitamin C, and the precursor to vitamin A, beta-carotene.

New information on these basic antioxidants is available since my previous book, but my recommendations on nutritional therapy and dosages remain substantially the same. (For the specific dose recommendations for men, women, and children in different age-groups and activity categories, see my *Antioxidant Revolution*, p. 127.)

Other nutrients are now emerging as powerful players in the antioxidant scenario. One of these, which we have already discussed in some detail in Chapters 2 and 3, is folic acid. I consider folic acid supplements and folate-rich foods to be a requirement. Other antioxidants, like selenium and coenzyme Q10, may have a beneficial impact, but they are still optional in my recommendations. But now let's turn to some of the new information we have about antioxidants.

THE ONGOING ANTIOXIDANT SAGA

President Richard Nixon declared a "War on Cancer" in his State of the Union address on January 22, 1971. But the results have been less than auspicious. In the twenty-five years since Nixon's declaration, the National Cancer Institute invested $29 billion in what some critics have called a "medical Vietnam."

Here's the reason for the criticism: In 1996, experts projected that 550,000 Americans would die from cancer—215,000 more than in 1971! By the year 2000, it's possible that the incidence of cancer will rise even more and overtake heart disease as the nation's number one killer.

The evidence for an increase in cancers and a failure of government attempts at research and prevention has been flooding in from other quarters. In a study conducted by the Office of the Assistant Secretary for Health, Dr. Devra Davis reported on the decreasing deaths from cardiovascular disease and the rising number of cancer deaths among whites in the United States from 1973 to 1987. She was able to show that, after adjustments were made for age and sex, there are considerably more cancer deaths now than there were among Americans born in an earlier era, from 1888 through 1897. Furthermore, there is more than twice as much cancer not linked to smoking as there was in the past. (See *JAMA*, February 9, 1994, pp. 431-7.)

Another study looked at the decline in semen quality among fertile men in Paris during the past twenty years. In 1973, the sperm count was 89 million per milliliter of semen in healthy, fertile men. But by 1992, the count had dropped to 60 million per milliliter—a level that is heading toward borderline infertility. (Any count above 60 million is considered good, while less than 20 million is considered infertile.) If this trend were to continue, in another forty years infertility might become a real problem in Paris, and perhaps elsewhere. (See *New England Journal of Medicine*, February 2, 1995, pp. 281-5.)

In both of the above studies, there are strong indications that these problems are due to something that has changed in our environment. One strong possibility is that the oxygen we breathe has been damaged by the pollution of our environment. This sort of damage would result in a proliferation of "free radicals"—unstable, destructive oxygen molecules—in our bodies.

How can we tell if too many free radicals are roaming about in our bodies? Since the publication of my *Antioxidant Revolution*, new technology has developed enabling us to measure more accurately free radical activity in our bodies. In the past, we measured "TBARS" as an indication of the by-products of free radical damage to blood vessels, which preceded the clogging of the arteries, but the results were neither reliable nor consistent. Now, another technology has developed—the measurement of F2 isoprostanes—which can give us a much more reliable indicator of free radical damage.

Dr. Jason Morrow of Vanderbilt University, Nashville, Tennessee, studied F2 isoprostane levels in smokers and nonsmokers, in an effort to ascertain free radical damage. He found the levels were considerably higher in smokers— a fact leading him to believe that some of the diseases associated with cigarette smoking, such as heart disease and lung cancer, may be directly related to free radical activity. (See *New England Journal of Medicine*, May 4, 1995, pp. 1198-203.)

An observation: If Morrow's conclusions are correct, some of the harmful effects of tobacco might be controlled by increasing the consumption of antioxidants in food and supplements.

To study further the effects of smoking and the protective effect of antioxidants, some investigators from the University of Freiburg, Germany, have measured forearm blood flow in smokers and nonsmokers. Drugs were infused into the artery supplying blood to the lower arm in an effort to dilate the vessel in both smokers and nonsmoking control subjects. Then, a large dose of vitamin C was infused into the arm.

The results? In the controls there was no change. But in the smokers there was marked improvement in forearm blood flow. (See *Circulation*, July 1, 1996, pp. 6-9.) This German finding supports the belief that oxygen-derived free radicals in chronic smokers are in part responsible for some of the vascular changes that lead to an increase in cardiovascular problems, such as heart attacks and strokes.

Again, the possibility of using antioxidants in controlling these diseases is intriguing.

The Starring Role of Fruits and Vegetables

As research continues into the antioxidant question, it becomes increasingly clear that the best way to get these free radical fighters is through your food. The main reason is that various vitamins, minerals, and other nutrients tend to work together, often in ways that scientists don't understand at the present time. So rather than rely primarily on tablets that may provide just one vitamin or mineral, it's best, whenever possible, to let nature provide you with a complete package.

Of course, there are limits to what you can take in through your food. Most likely, supplements will always have a place in a complete nutritional program, especially in helping us get adequate amounts of vitamin E and even vitamin C. But the more of these nutrients you can get through your diet, the better.

For example, it has been proven that there is a protective effect of fruits and vegetables against the development of strokes in men. For more than twenty years, Dr. Matthew Gillman, as part of the famous Framingham study, followed 832 men, ages forty-five to sixty-five, all of whom began the study free of cardiovascular disease. He conducted this study to evaluate the well-known observation that countries with high fruit and vegetable intake have low stroke rates.

At the end of his investigation, he determined that for every increase of three servings of fruit or vegetables a day, there was a 22 percent decrease in the risk of all strokes. In other words, "an increase in three fruits and vegetables a day may indeed keep stroke away!" (See *JAMA*, April 12, 1995, pp. 1113-7.)

In an interview in the *Journal of the American Medical Association*, Dr. Bruce Ames, professor of biochemistry and molecular biology and director of the National Institute of Environmental Health Sciences Center at the University of California, Berkeley, summed up the situation this way:

> The beneficial effects of fruit and vegetable consumption are so large when it comes to health.
> People in the bottom quartile of dietary intake of fruits and vegetables have twice the cancer rate for most types of cancer as people in the top quartile. People in the top quartile were consuming in the range of the two fruits and three vegetables we should be eating every day. . . .
> The rates of heart disease and cataracts are much higher in people not eating enough fruits and vegetables. I think all of the degenerative diseases of aging will be minimized by a good diet. . . .
> At the moment, we haven't identified all the compounds in foods that have antioxidant properties or which foods may have the highest levels of these compounds. Eventually we will. But that's why some people feel that you shouldn't just be taking vitamins without eating fruits and vegetables. (*JAMA*, April 12, 1995, pp. 1077-8.)

This expert opinion further confirms the importance of getting as much of your antioxidant intake as possible from food sources. As Dr. Ames indicates, we are still in a relatively early stage of research into how specific nutrients can affect human health. More and more, scientific studies suggest that an entire item of food, such as a cruciferous vegetable or a citrus fruit, is preferable to the tiny "piece" of that food found in a particular vitamin or mineral supplement. The whole nutritional "package" of a food item seems to deliver the most benefit.

This advice applies more to vitamin C and beta-carotene than it does to vitamin E. It is quite possible for many people to get their full complement of vitamin C and beta-carotene by eating at least five to seven helpings of fruits and vegetables every day. But don't worry if you fall short in reaching the minimum through your foods. You can take supplements to make up the difference. That way, you will be sure to reach the recommended minimums I have indicated in my recommendations for the two nutrients.

As for vitamin E, it's virtually impossible to take in a sufficient amount through the diet—at least 400 international units (IU) per day. So you should plan on taking at least 400 IU per day of vitamin E in the form of supplements.

Note: For more on this issue, including a listing of grams of vitamin C, beta-carotene, and vitamin E in specific foods, see chapter 7 of my *Antioxidant Revolution*. Also, refer to the "Vitamin C," "Vitamin A," and "Vitamin E" entries in Part II of this book.

Vitamin E—The Antioxidant Powerhouse

The evidence is building that vitamin E should be the cornerstone of an antioxidant therapy program.

In an interview in *Runner's World* (March 1996, p. 22), the world-renowned expert on antioxidants, Dr. Barry Halliwell, rated vitamin E as the antioxidant with the "most promise."

A great deal of evidence supports Halliwell's conclusion. For example, in the March 30, 1996, issue of the British medical journal *Lancet*, researchers from Northwick Park Hospital in London reported that daily doses of vitamin E, taken by people with bad hearts, can reduce heart attacks by 75 percent. The benefits of taking vitamin E to reduce the risk of a nonfatal heart attack became evident after about 200 days of treatment, indicating the importance of the cumulative effect of the vitamin.

Even Dr. Nigel Brown, the leader of the study, was

amazed at the findings. "We were surprised by the magnitude of the result," he said, "but it does seem to be true." (See *Palm Beach Post*, March 26, 1996, p. 6A.)

In other recent research results, vitamin E's reputation for cardiovascular protection has been extended.

- Vitamin E intake of 100 IU per day or more has been shown to reduce the progress of coronary artery lesions, according to scientists from the University of Southern California. In other words, vitamin E can actually slow the clogging of arteries that occurs with atherosclerosis. (See *Journal of the American Medical Association*, June 21, 1995, pp. 1849-54.)
- Taking 900 IU of vitamin E daily for four months lowered "bad" LDL cholesterol in thirty elderly, moderately obese men and women with stable angina (chest pains resulting from heart problems). Also, this study showed indirect evidence that LDL oxidation (damage to "bad" LDL cholesterol from free radicals) was reduced after the vitamin E intake. (See *American Journal of Clinical Nutrition* report cited in *Nutrition & the M.D.*, July 1995, p. 8.)
- In two related, long-term studies of thousands of men and women by the Harvard School of Public Health, researchers determined that taking at least 100 IU of vitamin E daily in supplements for at least two years is associated with a lower risk of heart disease in both men and women. (See *New England Journal of Medicine*, May 20, 1993, pp. 1444-56.)

Other recent studies show that cardiovascular benefits are only the beginning of the vitamin E story.

Researchers reporting in 1995 in *Mutation Research* found a significant increase in DNA damage in the cells of people who took no supplements, twenty-four hours after they had exercised. But those who took 800 IU of vitamin E three times—twelve hours and two hours before exercise, and again twenty-two hours after exercise—experienced reduced DNA strand breakage.

Furthermore, when the subjects were given 1,200 IU of vitamin E for fourteen days prior to exercise, their DNA damage was reduced even further. In fact, in four out of five participants, the vitamin E supplements completely prevented DNA damage after exhaustive exercise. *Note:* DNA and other cell damage have been linked to cancers of various types.

How much vitamin E should you be taking to get the full benefits? Although some of the above studies showed significant results with only 100 IU per day, I'm inclined to agree with a report by Dr. Ishwarlal Jialal, who conducted a 1995 study at the University of Texas Southwestern Medical Center in Dallas. He saw reductions in oxidized LDL cholesterol in the blood beginning with doses of 400 IU per day.

Therefore, I would regard 400 IU as the bottom line for daily dosage. Of course, even higher doses should be taken by those who are heavy exercisers, who weigh more than 200 pounds, or who are in other high-risk categories. (See my specific recommendations on page 127 of *Antioxidant Revolution*.)

In spite of the great publicity that vitamin E has received, it's important to keep in mind that there are other important players in basic antioxidant therapy—namely, vitamin C and beta-carotene. I say this even though both of these nutrients have encountered some skepticism and have been the center of controversies in recent years.

The Rehabilitation of Beta-Carotene

Several studies of the dietary intake of beta-carotene have shown it to be *inversely* related to cardiovascular disease. That is, the more beta-carotene you consume, the lower your risk of heart and artery problems. (But smoking may wipe out this benefit, according to some studies.)

The cardiovascular benefits of beta-carotene were also supported by the Coronary Primary Prevention Trial (LUC-CPPT). Dexter Morris and his colleagues followed 1,899 men, ages forty to fifty-nine, who for the previous thirteen years had no known preexisting coronary heart disease, cancer, or other major illness. Those men with higher total blood serum carotenoid levels had a *decreased* risk of coronary heart disease. Again, this benefit was stronger among men who never smoked.

Reducing the risk of cardiovascular disease is not the only established benefit of beta-carotene. In Americans over sixty-five years of age, macular degeneration of the eye is the leading cause of blindness. Dr. Johanna Seddon and colleagues compared 356 people with advanced stages of macular degeneration with 520 control subjects. A higher dietary intake of carotenoids was clearly associated with a lower risk of macular degeneration. The specific carotenoids included leutin and zeoxanthin, which are primarily obtained from dark green, leafy vegetables, such as spinach and collard greens. (See *JAMA*, November 9, 1994, pp. 1413-20.)

Yet beta-carotene has come under attack in the popular press as a result of several studies, including a 1994 report on Finnish smokers, and an investigation known as the "Beta-Carotene and Retinol Efficacy Trial (CARET)." In these reports, lung cancer actually increased in the smokers taking beta-carotene. For more specifics on these and related reports, see the entry "Vitamin A" in Part II of this book.

The negative conclusions about beta-carotene that are being drawn from these studies are flawed for a couple of reasons. First, the studies thought to be most damaging to beta-carotene deal only with high-risk patients—cigarette smokers.

Second, the increase in death rates linked to beta-carotene was not "statistically significant." In other words, more extensive studies with a larger population sample need to be conducted before we can come to any final conclusions.

Third, it is well documented that people whose blood level of beta-carotene is high have the lowest risk of death from all causes. The problem is that supplemental beta-carotene does not always increase blood levels of the nutrient, possibly because of problems with absorption. This may be the reason why no beneficial effect of beta-carotene can be seen in cigarette smokers; that is, they may have special difficulties with absorption.

In a related development, Dr. Charles Hennekens and colleagues from Harvard Medical School followed 22,071 male physicians for twelve years in an effort to determine beneficial or harmful effects of beta-carotene. At the beginning of the study, the volunteers, who were forty to eighty-four years of age, included 11 percent current smokers and 39 percent former smokers. The participants took either a placebo or fifty milligrams (80,000 IU) of beta-carotene every day.

The results: Supplementation with beta-carotene produced neither benefit nor harm in terms of the incidence of cancer, heart disease, or deaths from all causes in either smokers or nonsmokers. (See *New England Journal of Medicine*, May 2, 1996, pp. 1145-9.)

It appears that in this highly significant, well-controlled study, beta-carotene supplements were not helpful; but they were certainly not harmful. Also, it's possible that the true effects of beta-carotene on the body may require more time than has been allotted in many of these studies.

For example, in an investigation reported in the *Journal of the American Medical Association* on March 6, 1996 (pp. 669-703), researchers found that daily supplementation with 80,000 IU of beta-carotene for an average 4.3 years didn't reduce deaths from cardiovascular disease, cancer, or other diseases. But in the 1,188 men and 532 women who were studied, mortality from all causes was approximately 40 percent lower among persons whose plasma beta-carotene concentrations were above average when they entered the study. In other words, these longer-lived people had higher levels of beta-carotene longer, and perhaps much longer than the 4.3-year duration of the study.

My current position on beta-carotene can be stated this way:

- To discourage beta-carotene consumption in low-risk patients (such as nonsmokers) is not yet warranted, because there are still a number of studies that show beneficial effects.
- Beta-carotene should never be used by heavy drinkers, and light drinkers should avoid taking beta-carotene four hours before and after drinking any alcohol.
- Generally speaking, it is best to get your beta-carotene and other carotenoids in their natural form. Eating five to seven daily servings of fruits and vegetables has proven effective in helping to prevent strokes, cancer, and cardiovascular disease.

The Vitamin C Controversy—A Tempest in a Teapot?

In a study reported by *The Proceedings of the National Academy of Sciences* on April 16, 1996, researchers from the National Institutes of Health (NIH) concluded that daily doses of vitamin C above 400 milligrams have no evident value. Also, they said that amounts of 1,000 milligrams or more may even be hazardous to health.

The researchers concluded that the optimum daily dose of vitamin C is probably around 200 milligrams. This recommendation contrasts with the much lower doses of 60 milligrams set as the Recommended Dietary Allowance (RDA), or the higher doses of 500 milligrams or more that I, and a number of other physicians and scientists, recommend.

In commenting on this study, some scientists have suggested that doses above 400 mg per day are not readily absorbed. In most cases, they say, the higher doses will quickly saturate the body's cells and blood with vitamin C. Because vitamin C is water-soluble, the excess is washed out of the body through the urine.

Also, some have worried about the danger of kidney stones or an overload of iron, which could be exacerbated by so much vitamin C. Yet, in my decades of dealing with thousands of patients taking high doses of vitamin C, I have never encountered one case of kidney stones, nor am I aware of any such studies in the literature.

I have several other questions about this NIH study. First of all, it focused on the effects of taking supplemental doses of the vitamin, not getting it through food intake. My own position is that most or all of your daily intake of vitamin C should come through your food.

Second, the study did not consider the effect of heavy perspiration that may accompany a high level of activity or stress. The more fluids and chemicals you lose through your sweat glands, the more you need to replenish your antioxidants, including vitamin C.

Third, no consideration was given to the known vitamin C deficiency usually seen in cigarette smokers. Because vitamins frequently are synergistic or interactive with other substances, any study looking at the beneficial or harmful effects of vitamin supplementation should first correct for such deficiencies.

Also, I wonder about the effect of extra body weight on vitamin C needs. I have recommended that those weighing more than 200 pounds should have higher doses of all the antioxidants because of their generally higher nutritional needs, and I still hold to that position.

Keep Your Eye on Coenzyme Q10 and Selenium

Researchers are building an increasingly compelling case for coenzyme Q10, which has been linked to prevention or treatment of a number of diseases associated with free radical damage. These include: protection of heart tissue after a heart attack, lowering of high blood pressure, help for congestive heart failure, reduction of irregular heartbeats, regression of breast cancer, and healing of periodontitis, or inflammation of the gums.

I cover this subject in some detail in the "Coenzyme Q10 (Ubiquinone)" entry in Part II, so I won't repeat myself here. Rather, I'll just say that no harm has been shown from taking doses of coenzyme Q10 up to 300 milligrams per day. You should regard this dosage as an optional, but not recommended, part of your personal antioxidant therapy.

The mineral selenium does seem to have an antioxidant effect, especially in protecting against oxidation of "bad" LDL cholesterol and some cancers. But the research reports at this point are mixed, and I still regard selenium as an optional part of your antioxidant arsenal. If you take it, limit your dosage to a maximum of 50 *micro*grams three times per day, and be aware of possible toxic effects from doses that approach or exceed 400 mcg per day. (The RDA for this mineral is 70 micrograms per day for men and 55 for women.) For more on this, see the "Selenium" entry in Part II.

A Warning for Heavy Exercisers

There is a general consensus that free radicals play an important role in the skeletal muscle damage that occurs after, or in conjunction with, strenuous exercise. The scientific literature suggests that dietary antioxidants, either in food or supplement form, are able to neutralize or detoxify some of these harmful effects.

Antioxidants produced within the body ("endogenous" antioxidants) also play a protective role. In trained athletes, the endogenous antioxidant activity increases markedly, and helps to control damage caused by free radicals (known as "oxidative stress"). So at least as far as free radical attacks are concerned, trained or fit individuals have an advantage over those who are untrained.

Physical training can even enhance our free radical defense system against the stress of moderate exercise, according to a study from Mahidol University in Thailand. Participants pedaled stationary bikes for an hour at 70 percent of their maximal effort. One group was relatively sedentary, while the other involved trained runners.

The researchers found that oxygen-containing free radicals increased in the blood of the sedentary subjects, but remained unchanged in the runners. They concluded that adaption to training in runners protects against possible muscle-damaging reactions. (See *Japanese Journal of Physical Fitness and Sports Medicine*, 1996, Vol. 45, pp. 63-70.)

But is there a point of diminishing returns with exercise?

For several years, my colleagues at the Cooper Aerobics Center and I have been studying the effects of very high levels of physical activity. To determine if there are harmful effects, we have looked at evidence of free radical damage in both the blood and urine. Measurement of the destruction of red blood cells (RBC lysis) is the best overall indicator of free radical activity. Also, F2 iso-prostanes are the best measure of "lipid peroxidation"—the oxidizing of LDL ("bad") cholesterol, which is the first step in the artery-clogging disease of arteriosclerosis. We have also measured the urine for DNA damage, which may be the first step in cancer.

Our studies show clearly that after being off any supplemental vitamins for six weeks or longer, nearly everyone loses protection against free radical damage. Yet in only six weeks, that protection can be brought back to normal with only modest supplements of vitamins C, E, or beta-carotene.

In light of these findings, I am not discouraging high levels of physical activity. But I am exercising caution about recommending strenuous activity unless the individual is consuming minimum doses of antioxidants as follows:

> 500 mg of vitamin C, twice a day
> 400 IU of vitamin E, once a day
> 25,000 IU of beta-carotene, twice a day

Individually or collectively, these vitamins seem to be very effective in controlling free radical damage. Also, scientific support for antioxidant supplements is increasing. One study has reported that runners taking daily supplements of vitamin C (250 mg), vitamin E (1,148 mg of alpha tocopherol equivalents), and beta-carotene (7.5 mg, or 12,500 IU) showed dramatically fewer signs of free radical damage than before they began taking the supplements. (See *Journal of Applied Physiology*, 1993, Vol. 74, pp. 905-9.)

We are still in the early stages of gathering scientific data on the dangers of heavy exercise and the value of antioxidant supplements. But bit by bit, an increasingly convincing case is being constructed.

For example, the *American Journal of Epidemiology* published a 1994 report on exercise and breast cancer, based on the famous Framingham Heart Study of more than 2,000 women. The researchers said that their findings did not support a protective effect of physical activity during adulthood for breast cancer. On the contrary, their data suggested an increased risk among more active women.

A scientific paper, presented by University of Washington scientists at the American Academy of Neurology and reported in the summer 1995 *AMAA Quarterly*, explored the possible link between amyotrophic lateral sclerosis (ALS), also called Lou Gehrig's disease, and vigorous exercise. ALS involves progressive muscle and spinal cord degeneration that eventually result in death.

This study established a connection between groups of laborers with ALS and their involvement in heavy physical activity. One possible explanation for the exercise-disease link was that the stress of overdoing physical work may generate free oxygen radicals that cause cellular damage and bring on the disease.

There is also a possible connection between free radicals and Parkinson's disease (PD). The mechanism may be free radicals produced in the brain. There have been preliminary reports that vitamin C and vitamin E may help reduce PD symptoms, or even hold back the progression of the disease. (See A. N. Lieberman and F. L. Williams, *Parkinson's Disease*, Simon & Schuster, 1993, p. 83.)

The increasing incidence of brain tumors is another indication that free radical damage may be on the rise. In the mid-1980s, about 55,000 Americans had brain tumors, according to national medical surveys. But in 1996, experts were predicting that the number would exceed 100,000.

On the clinical level, I have now assembled more than 150 cases of elite athletes who have developed classic free radical-related diseases. These include: brain tumors, other cancers, Parkinson's disease, Alzheimer's disease, and premature heart disease.

Here is a sampling from my files:

- James Livermore, a seasoned marathoner who ran the distance in less than three hours, developed heart problems and suffered a nonfatal heart attack at age forty-seven.
- Preston Moore, another experienced marathoner, passed out during a training run at a blistering 6:30 minutes-per-mile pace. He developed a serious heart irregularity, which is now controlled with medication. Also, a parathyroid tumor (on the gland located on the neck) was discovered during his medical checkup.
- Marshall Sessions, another dedicated marathoner, developed Parkinson's disease after running many demanding races. He trained by running forty to fifty miles per week.
- Orville Rogers, an airline pilot, ran many marathons and set the record in our clinic for a treadmill performance in his age category. But he developed heart disease and had to undergo a multivessel bypass operation. The problem was clogged arteries, a likely result of oxidized "bad" LDL cholesterol. Today, Orville is leading a normal life because he is on medication to control his cholesterol.
- Graham Farquharson, a Canadian businessman, was an extremely active athlete in his early fifties. He worked out at least five days a week in a number of sports, running 10-kilometer distances, playing hockey, running on a treadmill, and doing weight training. On one occasion, he organized a marathon to be run north of the Arctic Circle. But then he developed a malignant nodule in the thyroid gland, which was successfully removed surgically.

These are by no means isolated cases. They fit right in with many of the elite athletes you read about in your newspaper:

- Steve Scott, the American record-holder for the one-mile run and the first American to run a sub-four-minute mile 100 times, was diagnosed and treated for testicular cancer.
- Tim Gullikson, professional tennis player and coach of top-ranked Pete Sampras, died of brain cancer in 1996 at the age of forty-four.
- Russian skating star and two-time Olympic champion Sergei Grinkov died of a blocked coronary artery in 1995 at the age of twenty-eight.
- Two-time Olympic 800-meter medalist Kim Gallagher was reported to be suffering from stomach cancer in 1995 and was told at that point that she had two to three years to live.
- Greg LeMond, the star American bicyclist who was a three-time Tour de France winner, retired in 1994 because of a rare muscular disease, mitochondrial myopathy. The mitochondria are the "power packs" in the body's cells that are responsible for energy production.

Of course, there is no proof that any of these tragic cases are the direct result of extremely demanding physical training, which produces excess numbers of free radicals. Nor is there any proof that antioxidant therapy would have prevented the problems. But the evidence is strong enough for me to remain firm in my recommendation that elite athletes and other strenuous exercisers should take extra antioxidants to protect themselves.

You have many reasons to increase your intake of antioxidants. To sum up, let me provide adult readers with these reminders:

- To maximize your health, you *must* take in a minimum of 400 IU of vitamin E per day, preferably through the natural type of supplements (d-alpha tocopherol). Those who are not on vitamin E supplements are just not informed about the proven health benefits.
- You *must* take in a minimum of 500 to 1,000 milligrams of vitamin C daily, preferably through foods high in vitamin C, though supplements are certainly acceptable if you can't get enough through your diet.
- You *must* take in a minimum of 25,000 IU of beta-carotene daily through your diet. Remember, one and a half medium-size carrots will provide you with all you need.

These, of course, are just the rock-bottom requirements for every adult. As I've indicated elsewhere, specific recommendations will vary depending on your age, activity level, and gender. But if you at least begin with these minimum amounts of antioxidants, you will be taking a giant step toward protecting yourself from a wide variety of serious diseases.

PART II

THE A TO Z OF NUTRIMEDICINE

Chapter 5

Learning the Alphabet of
Nutritional Therapy

Many foods and nutrients
may be used for "nutritional therapy" in the broad sense
that they contribute to overall good health, bodily growth,
and improved energy. But certain foods, supplements, and
other nutrients have also developed the *specific* reputation
of being able to accomplish *particular* health goals.

For example, in some cases specific vitamins or groups
of vitamins, such as folate, the B-complex vitamins, or the
antioxidant vitamins C, E, and beta-carotene, have been
linked to a decreased incidence of serious conditions such
as cancer and heart disease. Other nutrients have been
associated with the relief or healing of troublesome problems like constipation, cataracts, skin diseases, lower
energy levels, depression, anxiety, and a lack of mental acuity.

What this means is that you can often "take" a food or
nutrient, much as you would take a medicine or prescription drug, and expect to enjoy improved health as a result.
The challenge is to identify the particular nutrient that will
help you with a particular problem, and then to know how

much of it your body requires. To maximize the health benefits, you must know your recommended nutritional "prescription."

THE A TO Z PRESCRIPTION

This second part of the book has been arranged alphabetically to enable you to use nutrients *prescriptively* to ward off specific physical and emotional health problems. The various entries have been selected to give priority to those with the greatest potential to further specific types of healing or achieve other health objectives.

In the following pages you will find certain nutrients that have little or no proven value for nutritional therapy. Yet, because they have been touted in the news media or have otherwise gained popularity, I believe they deserve some mention, even if I am neutral about them or recommend against their use.

The references in this part, which you can also access through the Contents at the beginning of the book, include a diversity of topics. The issues run the gamut from health complaints, to foods that are particularly important in therapy, to supplements and, finally, to special nutrients.

Despite this wide range of subject matter, most of the entries fit naturally into this simple format:

- First, you will see a brief introduction to the entry.
- Next, you will find a section called "Basic Nutritional Therapy." Here, I include the scientific basis for using particular foods or nutrients to prevent or heal disease. Also, I offer a basic approach to the therapy.
- Following this is a section labeled "Extra Scientific Information." Under this heading are the very latest research findings, as well as other relevant scientific studies.

- The "Special Food Sources, Strategies, and Facts" sections vary in content, depending on whether the main topic is a health condition, a food, a supplement, or a nutrient. For example, where the entry focuses on a food like meat, you will find a discussion of how lean steak might be used strategically by some people to raise their low levels of "good" cholesterol (high density lipoprotein or HDL) in the blood. In contrast, with a nutrient or supplement like beta-carotene (under the general heading "Vitamin A and Its Relatives"), the nutrient's food sources, such as apricots, carrots, and sweet potatoes, will be highlighted. With a topic like alcohol, the focus may be on special facts, such as how specific amounts of alcoholic beverages have been shown to have certain health benefits or risks.
- Every entry also contains my own "Therapy Recommendations," including the daily amounts of helpful supplements or quantities of certain foods.
- At the end of the entry I provide some cross-references to help you find other information on the particular issue.

Here is an example of how this A to Z section works:

Suppose you are middle-aged or older, and you have started to worry about deterioration or loss of your eyesight. If you look under the entry for "Eye Complaints," you will find a reference for a condition called "Age-Related Macular Degeneration," or AMD, which is the leading cause of blindness for people over sixty-five. You will then be cross-referenced to an expanded discussion of the topic under "Vitamin A and Its Relatives."

As you read, you will discover that a study reported in the *Journal of the American Medical Association* in November 1994 revealed that the way to prevent this problem may be to eat plenty of dark, leafy vegetables, such as spinach and collard greens. Cross-references to this study will also be found in the index under "Lutein" and "Zeaxanthin," the nutrients believed to help ward off AMD.

Or, take another example: You may be a big believer in the antioxidant mineral selenium. But when you look under "Selenium" in this A to Z section, you find that there is currently little scientific backing for taking this nutrient as a special supplement. It's true that some animal studies show that high doses can protect against cancer, but the results on humans have been inconclusive. In fact, a Harvard study published in April 1995 in the *Journal of the National Cancer Institute* found that higher levels of selenium did not protect women against breast cancer.

So, under the selenium "Therapy Recommendations," I say that I continue to be cautious about suggesting selenium supplements as a form of nutritional therapy. Instead, I conclude that taking supplements up to 150 micrograms a day should be regarded as optional.

HOW TO READ THIS BOOK

Many of my readers and patients love to read all of every popular medical book they buy, because they have a voracious appetite for expanding their knowledge about personal health issues. However, don't assume that to get the most out of Part II you have to read all the entries in order. Instead, you may want to glance over the Contents and check those items that relate to particular health concerns or to foods or supplements that may already be part of your nutritional program.

With this volume on your family health bookshelf, you can use it as questions arise about your nutritional program. And you can be sure that such questions will arise on a regular basis as you conduct your ongoing personal investigation of new foods and scientific findings. You will discover, as I have, that there is no substitute for a professionally designed, scientifically proven research aid such as this systematic A to Z guide to the health impact of specific foods, nutrients, and supplements on various diseases and medical conditions.

Chapter 6

Nutrimedicine from A to Z

VITAMIN A AND ITS RELATIVES

Vitamin A and its "relatives," including the carotenoids, such as beta-carotene, have a variety of important uses in healing and preventive medicine. If you use supplements, it's extremely important to know exactly what type of vitamin A-related substance you are dealing with and also the medical implications of using it. Otherwise, you could actually find yourself facing a serious threat to your health. (See discussion under "Basic Nutritional Therapy.")

Basic Nutritional Therapy

Vitamin A (retinol) plays an important role in maintaining the quality and health of your eyesight, skin, teeth, bones, and mucous membranes—the mucus-producing cells that line such bodily surfaces as the nasal passages, respiratory tract, vagina, and intestines. Also, vitamin A assists in the growth and repair of body tissues and may bolster your resistance to infection. As an antioxidant, high blood levels of beta-carotene (a precursor to vitamin A) have been linked to a reduction in the risk of lung cancer.

But there is also a downside to this nutrient. Vitamin

A can be toxic if you allow too much to enter your body, especially through vitamin A supplements or even excess consumption of vitamin A from animal foods.

You can usually get all the vitamin A you need through your meals, and I certainly suggest that you include plenty of vitamin A-rich foods in your diet (see "Food Sources"). But I do *not* recommend that you take any vitamin A supplements unless your physician specifically prescribes them!

In patients taking daily doses higher than 5,000 to 10,000 international units (IU), symptoms of vitamin A overdose may occur, including: blurred vision, hair loss, nausea, and dry skin. In the most severe cases, there may also be damage to the liver, birth defects, and enlargement of the spleen. But except for birth defects, which may result from women taking over 10,000 IU per day during pregnancy, serious vitamin A problems tend to occur after a person has taken 50,000 IU a day for many years.

Beta-carotene, a chemical precursor of vitamin A, presents a somewhat different picture. This substance, which is transformed into vitamin A after it enters the body, is part of the "carotenoid" family of nutrients. Their pigments are the source of the yellow, orange, and green colors in certain vegetables and fruits, like carrots, cantaloupe, sweet potatoes, spinach, collard greens, and kale.

Higher blood serum levels of beta-carotene have been linked to a lower risk of cataracts, heart disease, and cancers, such as rectal cancer, melanoma, and bladder cancer. But the question is, how do you increase the amounts of this nutrient in your blood?

The best way to take beta-carotene into your body is through foods high in this nutrient, such as carrots and sweet potatoes. Recent studies have cast doubt on the benefits of getting beta-carotene through supplements.

Generally speaking, beta-carotene supplement doses

below 50,000 IU (30 milligrams) per day should produce no serious side effects in most people, with three possible exceptions: smokers, heavy drinkers, and pregnant women.

In fact, two studies, one involving Finnish smokers published in the *New England Journal of Medicine* in April 1994, and a second reported at a press conference by the National Cancer Institute in January 1996, have suggested a link between megadoses of beta-carotene and an increased risk of deaths from lung cancer and heart disease for smokers.

The meaning of these studies isn't really clear. For one thing, the researchers conceded that the increased risks for smokers associated with beta-carotene were "not statistically significant." So the negative results for beta-carotene should not be given too much weight.

Also, participants in the 1996 report of the study involving smokers, which is known as the "Beta-Carotene and Retinol Efficacy Trial," took in large doses of vitamin A supplements along with the beta-carotene. As a result, the extent to which the health problems of the smokers were due to the vitamin A, as opposed to the beta-carotene, is unclear.

Still, the institute scientists noted that the negative effects on smokers were sufficiently worrisome to warrant taking smokers in the study off all their supplements, including beta-carotene.

The other 1996 study, the Physicians' Health Study, focusing on more than 22,000 doctors who took 50 milligrams of beta-carotene every other day, found that the beta-carotene supplements, while not harmful to nonsmokers, did not protect them against cancer or heart disease. In other words, the supplements appeared to be neutral in their effect for this group.

In light of these findings, Dr. Richard Klausner, director of the National Cancer Institute, which financed the two studies, has recommended against taking any beta-carotene supplements.

My own feeling, which I have expressed in other contexts, is that it's best to get your beta-carotene from foods that are high in the nutrient, such as carrots, sweet potatoes, cantaloupe, and mangoes. Beta-carotene supplements up to about 25,000 IU a day should be regarded as optional, or a second line of defense.

Finally, beta-carotene may have another, less serious side effect: Higher doses may cause a yellowish cast to the skin. This condition poses no real health threat, but does need to be considered from a cosmetic point of view.

Other carotenoids may produce specific health benefits. One study published in November 1994 in the *Journal of the American Medical Association* concluded that the carotenoids lutein and zeaxanthin, typically found in dark, leafy greens like spinach and collards, can provide protection from blindness in older people.

This study, conducted by Dr. Johanna H. Seddon of the Harvard Medical School and several colleagues, found that patients over age sixty-five who consumed the two types of greens five to six times a week had a 57 percent lower chance of getting "age-related macular degeneration," or AMD, than did those who consumed the smallest amounts of the greens. Foods rich in beta-carotene, such as carrots, did not produce any special benefits in warding off AMD.

Why should dark green, leafy vegetables be so effective with AMD? The researchers speculated that the carotenoids lutein and zeaxanthin, so abundant in those foods, may protect the retina from the damaging effects of blue light.

There is still more to the carotenoid story. Another member of this nutritional family, lycopene, which is found in tomatoes and gives them their red color, has been linked to lower rates of prostate cancer. A six-year study published in December 1995 in the *Journal of the National Cancer*

Institute revealed that men of southern European ancestry, from countries such as Italy and Greece, were the most likely to eat tomato-based products and the least likely to develop prostate cancer.

More specifically, researchers have found that tomato sauce is most strongly linked to a lower prostate cancer risk. The next best foods, in descending order of importance, are: raw or cooked tomatoes, pizza, and tomato juice. Green, leafy vegetables, fruits, and other common cancer-protective foods fail to lower the prostate cancer risk.

One of the researchers in this study, Dr. Edward Giovannucci of the Harvard School of Public Health, concluded that the more tomatoes you consume, the better. Those in the study with the lowest incidence of prostate cancer ate at least ten servings a week of tomato-based foods.

Extra Scientific Information

- Among babies born to women who took more than 10,000 IU of "preformed" or fully formed vitamin A (retinol) per day in the form of supplements, about one infant in fifty-seven had a malformation, including defects in the cranial (skull) tissue. (See *New England Journal of Medicine*, November 23, 1995, pp. 1369-73.)
- Vitamin A deficiency is one of the five major malnutrition problems in the world, and is most commonly found in children under the age of five. (See *Clinical Pharmaceutics*, 1993, Vol. 12, p. 506.) Children with this deficiency have a higher susceptibility to infections, diarrhea, and increased mortality.
- Infants with a respiratory virus infection were found to have lower blood serum levels of vitamin A in a study conducted at the Vanderbilt University School

of Medicine. The virus-infected children were then treated with high doses of oral vitamin A (12,500 to 25,000 IU), and their serum levels of the vitamin became normal, without any toxic effects. (See the May 1995 issue of *Antimicrobe Agents Chemotherapy*, pp. 1191-3.)

- High doses of vitamin A may reduce deaths from lung problems that result from the measles. In hospital-based studies, 80 percent of all measles-related deaths were due to respiratory infections. Vitamin A therapy reduced mortality by about 70 percent among patients who developed pneumonia, either before or after admission. (See *JAMA*, 1993, Vol. 269, p. 898.)

Currently the dose recommended by the World Health Organization (WHO) for treating measles is 100,000 IU of vitamin A for children younger than twelve months, and 200,000 IU in children older than twelve months. They take the doses by mouth.

- Very high doses of vitamin A reduced the incidence of sickness, especially diarrhea, among children born to HIV-infected women in Durban, South Africa.

Those who received the supplements were given 50,000 IU of vitamin A at one and three months of age; 100,000 IU at six and nine months; and 200,000 IU at twelve and fifteen months. The researchers, who were from the University of Natal in Durban, concluded that vitamin A supplementation for the children of these HIV-infected women appeared to be beneficial, probably because they were already suffering from vitamin A deficiencies. (See *American Journal of Public Health*, August 1995, pp. 1076-81.)

- Symptoms of soft tissue rheumatism can become worse if patients ingest an excessive amount of vitamin A. (See *West Virginia Medical Journal*, May 1995, p. 147.)

Special Food Sources, Strategies, and Facts

*   *Vitamin A sources:* dairy products such as milk and yogurt, cheese, eggs, liver, fish liver oil, and butter.
*   *Beta-carotene sources:* yellowish orange and green vegetables and fruits, including apricots, broccoli, cantaloupe, carrots, mangoes, papaya, spinach, sweet potatoes, and turnip greens.
*   *Lutein and zeaxanthin sources:* dark, leafy greens, such as spinach, collards, kale, mustard greens, and turnip greens.
*   *Lycopene sources:* tomatoes and tomato products such as tomato sauce, pizza containing tomatoes, watermelon, red grapefruit, and guava.

Cautionary fact: Be wary of the food additive olestra, which, according to some reports, dramatically reduces the body's ability to absorb carotenoids.

This additive, which has recently been approved by the U.S. Food and Drug Administration (FDA), is intended for use in potato chips and other snack foods as a fat substitute. But the foods with olestra carry a warning that it may cause abdominal cramping, loose stools, and poor absorption of some vitamins and other nutrients like beta-carotene.

Dr. Walter Willett, Chairman of the Nutritional Department at the Harvard School of Public Health, has cautioned that the effects of olestra may be linked to cancer, heart disease, and blindness. Also, Michael F. Jacobson, executive director of the Center for Science in the Public Interest, warns that as little as one ounce of olestra in potato chips could reduce carotenoid levels in the blood by 50 percent.

Therapy Recommendations

Avoid vitamin A supplements, but eat plenty of foods containing vitamin A, so long as those foods don't violate other important dietary principles such as maintaining a low-fat diet. For example, you should try to get your vitamin A from dairy products made from skim milk rather than whole milk.

Consume plenty of foods containing the carotenoids beta-carotene, lutein, zeaxanthin, and lycopene. (For a list of IU values of beta-carotene in different foods, see my *Antioxidant Revolution*, p. 148.)

So long as you are taking in at least 25,000 IU a day of beta-carotene from these foods, you can forget about taking any supplements. As a general rule, if you are a nondrinker, a nonsmoker, or a woman who is not pregnant, you may regard beta-carotene supplements as an optional part of your diet. But if you are pregnant, a smoker, or a moderate to heavy drinker, it is advisable that you do not take beta-carotene supplements.

By "moderate drinker," I mean that you drink more than one ounce per day of pure alcohol, but less than four ounces. One ounce translates into two 4-ounce glasses of wine, two beers, or one mixed drink.

This recommendation becomes even more imperative if you are a heavy drinker who takes in four ounces or more of pure alcohol per day. Animal studies have shown serious liver damage can result from the combination of beta-carotene supplements and high doses of alcohol. Even if you are a light drinker who takes in less than one ounce of pure alcohol per day, it's advisable not to take beta-carotene supplements within four hours before or after you have a drink.

Finally, vitamin A requirements may be lower in the elderly because they have a decreased ability to clear the vitamin through the liver and other tissues. Also, they may have an increased absorption of vitamin A through the gastrointestinal tract. Consequently, the elderly will probably need less of this vitamin.

Cross-References

See "Cancers," "Eye Complaints," "Heart Disease," "Olestra."

ALCOHOL

My advice has always been—and continues to be—that it's best to avoid all alcoholic beverages. However, a number of potential health benefits from light drinking have surfaced in the medical literature in recent years, and these are worthy of mention.

Basic Nutritional Therapy

For a number of years, researchers have known that alcohol can raise a person's levels of "good" cholesterol, or high-density lipoproteins (HDLs). Having relatively high HDLs—above 50 to 60 mm/dl for men and above 63 to 74 mm/dl for women—can provide excellent protection from atherosclerosis, the clogging of the arteries that produces so many heart attacks.

One problem with this use of alcohol, however, is that certain studies reveal that drinking may raise only one component in your HDLs, and that component may not be protective against heart disease.

Despite this limitation, a number of studies have taken the next step to show that *light* drinking can actually lower the risk of heart attacks. The Nurses' Health Study published in May 1995 in the *New England Journal of Medicine* concluded that light drinking for women, defined as about one to three mixed drinks of average alcoholic strength per week, can save lives by reducing the risk of heart disease.

Specifically, women who consumed one to three drinks a week had a 17 percent lower death rate than nondrinkers. A similar study in 1993 confirmed substantially the same results for men.

Warning: The above study of nurses found that those who consumed two or more drinks a day had a 19 percent higher risk of death than did the teetotalers.

These and other scientific reports caused the federal government to acknowledge officially for the first time in January 1996 that alcoholic beverages can be healthful. The newly released *Dietary Guidelines for Americans*, published every five years by the U.S. Department of Agriculture and the Department of Health and Human Services, said that benefits may accompany moderate consumption of alcohol with meals. You should interpret "moderate" in this context to mean no more than three mixed drinks a week for women and no more than one mixed drink a day for men. (See "Special Food Sources, Strategies, and Facts.")

But there was a word of caution. These agencies warned that higher levels of drinking could raise the risk of high blood pressure, stroke, heart disease, certain cancers, cirrhosis of the liver, birth defects, suicides, violence, and accidents.

Extra Scientific Information

- Low to moderate intake of wine was associated with lower mortality from cardiovascular (heart vessel) and cerebrovascular (brain vessel) disease, according to a study at the Danish Epidemiology Science Centre in Copenhagen. In contrast, a similar intake of spirits (hard liquor) was associated with an increased risk of these diseases. Beer drinking in this study had no effect on mortality. (See Gronbaek, M., et al., "Mortality associated with moderate intakes of wine, beer, or spirits," *British Medical Journal*, May 6, 1995, pp. 1165-9.)

- Adolescents who drink beer and spirits tend to be heavier drinkers and are more rebellious than those who drink wine exclusively, according to research done at the Addiction Research Foundation in Toronto. (See Smart, R. G., and Walsh, G. W., "Do some types of alcoholic beverages lead to more problems for adolescents?" *Journal of Studies of Alcohol*, January 1995, pp. 35-8.)
- Because most responses to alcohol in both humans and animals are inherited, an important part of future management or prevention of alcoholism and alcohol abuse may be gene therapy, according to a study at the Department of Medical Psychology, Oregon Health Sciences University. (See Buck, K. J., "Strategies for mapping and identifying quantitative trait loci specifying behavioral responses to alcohol," *Alcohol Clinical Experimental Research*, August 1995, pp. 795-801.)
- Dr. Walter Willett of the Harvard School of Public Health says that "avoiding too much alcohol is one thing women can do to reduce their breast cancer risk." He is convinced that there is an increased risk with as little as one drink a day. "At two or three drinks a week," he says, "the effect—if any—is low."

Other researchers have found that there is a 10 percent increase in risk for women who have one drink a day, compared to nondrinkers, and a 20 percent increase at two drinks a day. For lifelong drinking, there is a 40 percent increase in women who average one drink a day, and a 70 percent increase with two daily drinks.

Yet only 4 percent of all breast cancers can be attributed to alcohol, says Matthew Longnecker, an epidemiologist at the National Institute of Environmental Health Sciences in Research, Triangle Park, North Carolina. "It's possible that something about drinkers, other than [their consumption of] alcohol, raises their risk," he says. (See *Nutritional Action Healthletter*, January/February 1996, p. 6.)

Special Food Sources, Strategies, and Facts

Keep in mind that one drink of wine refers to one 4-ounce glass of wine; the alcohol content in most table wines is the same. Similarly, one bottle or can of beer has about as much alcohol as the next. But if you prefer spirits or mixed drinks, be sure to measure as precisely as possible the alcohol content of your drinks.

Remember, for men the goal is less than 1 ounce a day of pure alcohol. This means no more than 1/2-1 ounce of 80-proof spirits in one mixed drink each day. Women should have no more than three such mixed drinks *per week.*

For men, if you prefer wine or beer, you should limit yourself to no more than ten 4-ounce glasses of wine or ten beers per week. For women, the goal is no more than six glasses of wine or six beers *per week.*

Therapy Recommendations

If possible, avoid all alcoholic beverages. My own practice has convinced me that the threats to health and life far outweigh the potential benefits. There are many other ways to decrease your risk of heart disease and other conditions. For example, aerobic exercise will raise HDL levels more effectively than alcohol for most people.

If you must drink, be sure to keep your consumption at a light level: less than ten drinks per week for men (consider a 4-ounce glass of wine, one beer, or one cocktail as one drink), or six drinks a week for women.

Under no circumstances should you use beta-carotene supplements if you are a heavy drinker. If you do, you could be increasing your risk of liver disease and other serious health conditions. Also, even if you are a light drinker, don't take these supplements within four hours before or after you consume alcohol.

Under no circumstances should children or teenagers drink.

Cross-References

See "Vitamin A," "Cholesterol Regulation," "Heart Disease."

ALFALFA

Alfalfa, also called "purple medic" and "lucerne," is mostly known as a plant used to make hay to feed cattle and sheep, but there are human uses for this food as well. Its history as a cultivated crop goes back to 1000 B.C. in the Middle East; now the United States is the largest producer in the world.

Alfalfa stalks, with all parts of the plant including the green leaves, contain about 16 percent protein and 8 percent of various minerals like potassium, magnesium, calcium, and iron. Also, this food contains vitamins A, E, D, and K in very small amounts.

Basic Nutritional Therapy

It is best not to overemphasize alfalfa in your diet.

There are claims, generally unsupported by scientific research, that alfalfa is a wonder food. It has been touted for relief of arthritis, ulcers of the intestine, hemorrhoids, high blood pressure, bad breath, constipation, and even cancer. Also, eight enzymes found in alfalfa have been associated with claims of better digestion and assimilation of food. Although in individual cases alfalfa may help with these conditions, there is no proof that it will help anyone. In fact, in some cases, as indicated in the following section, too much may hurt.

Extra Scientific Information

- Alfalfa pills or diets high in alfalfa seed or sprouts have been associated with a higher incidence of the autoimmune disease, systemic lupus erythematosus (SLE), according to letters written by N. R. Farnsworth to the November 1995 issue of the *American Journal of Clinical Nutrition*. Also, inactive SLE may be activated by alfalfa tablets.
- Alfalfa sprouts were linked to a ten-state outbreak of "salmonella stanley," according to a report in the June 23, 1995 *Chicago Tribune*. Seventeen residents of the Chicago area were hit with this bacterial disease, which can cause headaches, fever, diarrhea, and vomiting. Four of these patients had to be hospitalized. According to the Centers for Disease Control in Atlanta, this risk of salmonella poisoning can be minimized if the alfalfa sprouts are washed thoroughly before they are eaten.
- Other studies have linked alfalfa to blood abnormalities and interference with the body's use of vitamin E.

Special Food Sources, Strategies, and Facts

If you enjoy the taste, feel free to include alfalfa sprouts in moderation as a topping or component for your salads, or to drink an occasional cup of alfalfa tea. But stay away from alfalfa tablets, since they may contain too high a dose of this legume.

Therapy Recommendations

The fiber and other nutrients in alfalfa can contribute to general good health. But at this point in our knowledge, it would be a mistake to think of the plant as a nutritional "magic bullet" capable of healing anything by itself.

Cross-References

See "Vitamin D," "Vitamin E," "Vitamin K."

ALLERGIES AND FOOD INTOLERANCES

For the most part, foods and nutrients will help heal or prevent various health problems. But in some cases the opposite may occur: Foods may actually trigger an allergic reaction. True food allergies are estimated to affect less than 2 percent of the population. About 5 percent of children have food allergies, which appear first in early childhood, but are frequently outgrown. Yet up to 40 percent of the general population believe they or a family member suffers from allergies to food. (See *Journal of Allergies and Clinical Immunology*, 1986, Vol. 78, p. 127.)

A food allergy, by definition, is any adverse reaction by the immune system to a generally harmless food or food ingredient. While nearly any food can cause an allergic response, the most common ones to which people are allergic are: eggs, fish, shellfish, soy products, red wines, Chinese food, wheat, peanuts, and tree nuts.

Non-immune-related reactions to food are known as "food intolerances," with lactose (milk sugar) intolerance being an example. Many people, especially as they grow older, find it harder and harder to tolerate dairy products because of bouts with stomach cramps, excessive gas, or diarrhea. This condition, known as "lactose intolerance," is caused by a lack of the enzyme lactase, which helps in the digestion of the milk sugar lactose.

Whether you are dealing with a true allergy or an intolerance, the challenge is to identify the offending food or nutrient and then take aggressive steps to prevent it from getting through your body's defenses.

Basic Nutritional Therapy

If you notice discomfort, pain, or other negative reactions after you eat certain foods, you may well have a food allergy or intolerance. Avoid eating the suspect food until you see your physician. Also, until you consult with your doctor, don't try any "home remedies" such as an elimination diet. An elimination diet involves trying and then omitting certain foods until you find the one that is causing the bad reaction. The reason for this caution is that, as the food is reintroduced, you could have such a severe reaction that eating it in any quantity could produce anaphylactic shock. This reaction can result in hives, internal swelling in the respiratory system, difficulties in breathing or inability to breathe, and even death.

Symptoms that may signal a food allergy or intolerance include: itching in the mouth, excessive gas, diarrhea, stomach cramps, hives, sneezing, watery eyes, swelling of the lips or other parts of the body, rashes, skin flushing, severe or migraine headaches, or difficulty in swallowing or breathing.

Extra Scientific Information

- Mustard that was "masked" in a chicken dip caused a severe anaphylactic reaction in a thirty-eight-year-old woman twenty minutes after she ate in a fast-food restaurant, according to the October 1995 issue of the *Annals of Allergy, Asthma, and Immunology*, pp. 340-2.
- Vomiting is a common symptom resulting from adverse food reactions in infants to such foods as cow's milk and soy milk. (See the August 1995 *Seminars of Pediatric Surgery*, pp. 147-51.)

- Peanuts are the most common cause of fatal and near-fatal food-induced anaphylaxis, according to the May 1995 issue of *Pediatric Allergy Immunology,* pp. 95-7.
- More children and adolescents die annually from food-induced anaphylaxis than from insect stings. (See the *Journal of the School of Nursing,* October 1995, pp. 30-2.)
- Eating a fresh fig triggered an anaphylactic reaction in a patient studied for *Allergy,* June 1995, pp. 514-6.
- Fresh kiwi caused an anaphylactic reaction in a fifty-seven-year-old man, and the same allergic response happened to a twenty-nine-year-old man who ate fish. (See *Allergy,* June 1995, pp. 511-3.)
- A woman who had developed an allergy to dust mites in her home experienced a severe allergic reaction after she ate snails. Researchers from the University Hospital, Utrecht, the Netherlands, surmised that the food allergy occurred because of initial sensitization by the dust mites. (See *Allergy,* May 1995, pp. 438-40.)
- People who are allergic to spices like coriander, caraway, paprika, cayenne, mustard, and white pepper also tend to be allergic to birch pollen and to at least one vegetable. (See *Annals of Allergy, Asthma, and Immunology,* September 1995, pp. 280-6.)
- Less than 1 percent of more than 3,000 adult patients studied in the Hospital de Amara, Guipuzcoa, Spain, tested positive for a food allergy, according to the *Journal of Investigative Allergology and Clinical Immunology* (January-February 1995, pp. 47-9). The most common offending foods were fresh fruit, dried fruits, seafood, and vegetables. The least common were chicken eggs.

- In a study conducted at the La Paz Children's Hospital, Madrid, Spain, 355 children were diagnosed with food allergies. The principal foods involved in allergic reactions were eggs, fish, and cow's milk. Other allergy-producing foods were peaches, hazelnuts, walnuts, lentils, peanuts, chickpeas, and sunflower seeds. Most of the patients (86.7 percent) reacted to only one or two foods, while 13.3 percent reacted to three or more foods (mostly to the legumes and fruits). (See *Pediatric Allergy Immunology*, February 1995, pp. 39-43.)
- A significant proportion of children with a cow's milk allergy experienced asthma when they ingested cow's milk, says a report in *Pediatric Pulmonology Supplement*, 1995, pp. 59-60.
- Though vegetable-induced asthma is uncommon, two unrelated vegetables, Swiss chard and green beans, were linked to acute asthma in a Spanish woman studied at the Hospital Ramon y Cajal, Madrid, Spain. (See *Annals of Allergy*, April 1993, pp. 324-7.)
- A three-year-old boy developed a severe anaphylactic shock reaction after eating a banana, and at the same time, showed hypersensitivity to contact with rubber (latex), according to an Italian study at the University of Verona. (See *Acta Paediatrica*, June 1995, pp. 709-10.)
- Barley flour may induce bronchial asthma through inhalation of allergens, reports the *Annals of Allergy, Asthma, and Immunology*, August 1995, pp. 121-4.
- A fifty-four-year-old woman developed episodes of asthma when she was exposed to the vapors from cooking certain kinds of legumes, including peas, chickpeas, beans, and lentils. (See *Allergology*

Immunopathology, January-February 1995, pp. 38-40.)

- Eliminating the offending food from the diet is the only proven therapy in confirmed cases of food allergy. In some cases, strict adherence to an elimination diet actually appears to promote the process of "outgrowing" an allergy, or developing tolerance to a food. But it may take one to two years of rigorously following an allergen-free diet. Allergies to peanuts, fish, and shellfish usually last a lifetime. (See *Journal of Pediatrics*, 1989, 115:23; *Journal of Allergies and Clinical Immunology*, 1989, 89:475.)

- A Maryland physician described symptoms he experienced after eating in a Chinese restaurant. He reported flushing; a burning sensation in the chest, neck, and abdomen; tightening of the jaw and upper chest muscles (which, at times, may make swallowing difficult); and headaches. These reactions occurred shortly after he ate foods containing monosodium glutamate (MSG), and they describe a condition that has come to be known as the "Chinese Restaurant Syndrome." (See *New England Journal of Medicine*, 1968, 278:1122.)

Special Food Sources, Strategies, and Facts

Here is a summary of some of the foods and nutrients that are most likely to produce particular allergic or intolerant reactions:

- Peanuts, tree nuts: associated with itching in the mouth, swelling, stomach pain and discomfort, breathing and swallowing problems.
- Shrimp, lobster, crabs, and other shellfish: may cause itching or swelling in the mouth, rashes, stomach pain, diarrhea, breathing and swallowing problems.

- Eggs: various allergic reactions, including anaphylactic shock.
- Milk and other dairy foods: abdominal cramps, gas, diarrhea.
- Fast-food hamburgers: sulfites used in hamburger food preparation, as well as in dried fruits, may cause severe headaches.
- Chinese food: additives, particularly MSG, may lead to hives, swelling, headaches, or fatigue.
- Fruits and vegetables, including those served at salad bars: chemicals used to spray these foods may trigger stinging, flushing, or other responses, even including asthma.
- Red wines: produce headaches in some people.

For more information, contact the Food Allergy Network, 4744 Holly Avenue, Fairfax, VA 22030; phone: (800) 929-4040.

Therapy Recommendations

If you know that every time you eat shrimp you have an allergic reaction, such as a swelling or itching in your mouth, then the obvious therapy is to avoid that food. On the other hand, if you are not sure of the offending food, you might try an elimination diet *under your doctor's or registered dietitian's supervision,* to help you identify it.

Elimination diets can be used both for diagnosis and for treating food allergies. Eliminate or restrict the suspected food from the diet for several weeks to determine if the current symptoms will subside. If improvement is seen, then the suspected food or foods may be introduced into the diet one at a time. Monitor whether symptoms recur. If they do, avoid the offending food in the future.

Note: Usually, an elimination diet will be all you need to find any problem you may have with food allergies and intolerances. But sometimes, other allergy tests administered by an allergy specialist, such as the "radioallergosorbent test," or RAST, may help ferret out food allergies.

Cross-References

See "Asthma," "Diarrhea."

AMINO ACIDS

Amino acids are smaller units, or "building blocks," that make up protein—the large molecules responsible for the growth and continuing health of our bodies, including muscles, ligaments, bones, hair, nails, enzymes, and hormones.

Of the more than twenty amino acids in our bodies, eight are considered "essential"; that is, the body cannot make them, so they must be taken in through the diet. These include isoleucine, leucine, lysine, methionine, phenylalanine, threonine, tryptophan, and valine. The others are known as "nonessential" amino acids because the body is able to synthesize them internally.

One way to remember this distinction is to recall the letter "E": essential amino acids must be *eaten*.

About 10 to 20 percent of the total calories consumed daily by the average adult should come from protein. No more than 20 to 30 percent should come from fats, and about 50 to 70 percent should come from complex carbohydrates like fruits and vegetables. This means that if you take in 2,000 calories a day, 200 to 400 of those calories should come from protein.

Here's an example of this from an average daily menu:

First, you should know that 1 gram of protein is equal to about 4 calories of energy. (For comparison's sake, be aware that 1 gram of carbohydrate also produces about 4 calories, while 1 gram of fat translates into 9 calories.) As you can see, on a 2,000-calorie diet, you would have to consume 50 to 100 grams of protein a day to get your 200 to 400 calories.

In a typical daily menu, 3½ ounces of chicken (light meat) contains about 30 grams of protein (4 calories per gram x 30 grams = 120 calories). Add to that a cup of skim milk for breakfast, and you get another 8 grams (32 calories) of protein. Finally, select one-half cup of bran cereal in the morning (4 grams or 16 calories of protein) and a cup of nonfat plain yogurt (12 grams or 48 calories of protein), and you will reach and move beyond your 200-calorie minimum daily need for protein.

Basic Nutritional Therapy

If you take in a reasonable variety of protein-containing foods, you will get the full range of amino acids you need. But there are two basic adjustments you should be ready to make if you want to maximize the benefits from these nutrients.

Protein adjustment 1: To get an adequate supply of amino acids, be sure to eat a variety of plant and animal protein products, including meats, grains, legumes, seeds, nuts, and vegetables.

Just as there are two basic types of amino acids, so there are also two categories of protein: complete and incomplete. Complete protein, which comes from animal-produced foods, such as beef, pork, chicken, fish, and dairy products, contains sufficient essential amino acids all by itself to contribute to the building of your muscle and other body tissues. In contrast, *in*complete protein, found in plant food such as vegetables, grains, nuts, seeds, and various beans, must be eaten in wide varieties to cover all the amino acids. Otherwise, they must be combined in your diet with some animal-produced protein (milk, cheese, or meat) to be maximally useful to your body.

So when your mother said, "Eat your peanut butter

sandwich," she was nutritionally correct. The incomplete protein in the peanut butter was made complete by combining it with the bread to provide all the essential amino acids.

Protein adjustment 2: Be ready to add extra amino acids through protein-rich foods when you feel you need them for special protection against certain health conditions.

In making this point, I am *not* suggesting that you load up on specialized amino acid or protein supplements. You can expect to get all the protein you need through your diet.

It is possible, however, to emphasize specific amino acids in your regular eating program in such a way that you *may* enhance particular health benefits. Here are some illustrations, using several amino acids that can have special effects in your body:

Reminder: As you move through these examples, remember that a "nonessential" amino acid is not an unnecessary one. Rather, the term refers to the fact that the body *can* produce that particular amino acid, while the body *cannot* produce an essential amino acid.

- *Arginine.* This nonessential amino acid has been linked to enhanced immunity, wound healing, and release of the growth hormone necessary for bodily growth in children and healing of damaged tissues. Some even say that arginine can increase a man's sperm count!

As with many other special nutrients and supplements, the claims for arginine often outrun the scientific findings.

Most research suggests that even though all amino acids affect growth hormone release to some extent, only arginine and ornithine have a significant effect. These are the amino acids usually sold to athletes as growth hormone promoters and muscle builders. Yet studies of arginine suggest that a minimum of 250 mg per kilogram of body weight is needed to stimulate growth hormone release. Most supplements contain only a few milligrams of arginine and will not affect hormone release. Ironically, this lack of an effect is fortunate in view of the known potential dangers of excess growth hormone. For most athletes, amino acid supplements are just expensive and unneeded, and I do not recommend their use.

There have also been claims that taking 3,000 to 6,000 mg of L-arginine daily will help reverse atherosclerosis. In addition, some say this supplement is essential for the promotion of nitric oxide, which promotes blood flow to the muscles. Furthermore, it's claimed that the supplement enhances muscle repair following exercise, as well as sexual potency. For the most part, however, this information is based on anecdotal reports, not documented in scientific journals.

Finally, pregnant women, nursing women, herpes sufferers, or schizophrenic patients may encounter special health complications with arginine supplements. (See "Extra Scientific Information.")

In general, taking *all* amino acids through the diet is the best idea, because you get a healthy combination of other nutrients and are unlikely to overdose on any one nutrient. (See the "Food Sources" section.)

- *Leucine.* One of the hottest supplements now on the market for muscle building by athletes is HMB, or "beta-hydroxy beta-methylbutyrate," a product that arises naturally from the metabolism of the essential amino acid leucine.

Some studies, particularly a 1995 investigation at Iowa State University, have reported that this product can accelerate the buildup of lean muscle tissues during strenuous exercise. In the well-designed, four-week study at Iowa State, 17 exercise-trained and 23 untrained men were divided into two groups: One took daily 3-gram supplements of HMB, and the other took placebo pills. Each group pursued the same weight lifting routine three times per week.

At the end of the study, the HMB group averaged a 3.1 percent increase in lean muscle mass, while the placebo group experienced only a 1.9 percent increase. Also, the HMB takers were able to bench-press 22 pounds more at the end of the study than they could at the beginning. In contrast, the placebo group increased their bench-press level by only 14 pounds. (See *American Medical News*, August 19, 1996, p. 17.)

The way HMB works in the body is still unclear, but researchers speculate that it may protect the body from tissue damage during heavy exercise. As a result, the body can redirect its energy from tissue repair to muscle building.

So far, no negative side effects have appeared with use of HMB supplements. In fact, those taking HMB have reported lower cholesterol and blood pressure levels. The main drawback at this point seems to be the cost; a week's supply sells for about $35. Also, more data is needed before I can give a recommendation.

Researchers at Iowa State and Vanderbilt caution that HMB, though apparently safe for men, should not be taken by children, pregnant women, or lactating women. Studies done on other women are still being analyzed.

- *Lysine.* This essential amino acid is especially important for the production of antibodies, hormones, and enzymes. Some people feel that this nutrient can help heal injuries, as well as relieve muscle strains and soreness.

The scientific research is not solid enough on these claims to warrant your taking special lysine supplements.

One exception is when lysine is combined with other vitamins and nutrients to create dietetic supplements that
increase the appetite of those who are anorexic or who need
to gain weight after an illness. However, such supplements
should be taken only under a physician's supervision. As
with other amino acids, it's best to rely on the protein in
your diet for lysine. (See "Food Sources.")

• *Phenylalanine.* Many alternative medicine enthusiasts believe that this essential amino acid can perform a variety of wonders, including improving
mental acuity, overcoming depression, suppressing
appetite (and thus enhancing weight loss), relieving
migraine headaches and various other pains, and
stimulating the sex drive. Whether it can produce
these effects has not been confirmed. But we do
know that phenylalanine has a special role in the
production of dopamine, epinephrine, and norepi-
nephrine—three chemical messengers.

Certain tablets containing high doses of the DL-phenyl-
alanine form of this nutrient can help correct amino acid
deficiencies in those who have problems with abuse of
alcohol, cocaine, and other drugs. Also, there are indications that these supplements can serve as an effective
painkiller.

But some strong medical warnings must be attached to
phenylalanine supplements. They can pose dangers to
pregnant or lactating females, growing children, and people
who are taking monoamine oxidase inhibitors (MAO),
which are used to treat depression in the elderly. Also, you
should definitely stay away from these supplements if you
have melanoma skin cancer, diabetes, or high blood pressure.

As with any other supplement, you should first have
your physician's approval before you take phenylalanine

tablets. Unless your doctor determines that you have a special need for supplements or medications containing this nutrient, stick to phenylalanine-rich foods! (See "Food Sources.")

- *Tryptophan.* Tryptophan is an essential amino acid that helps the brain produce the neurotransmitter serotonin, one of the chemicals that regulate the transmission of nerve impulses in the brain. Also, it is one of the major chemicals governing mood and behavior. The antidepressant drug Prozac works by increasing the serotonin levels in the brain.

This amino acid has been linked to such health benefits as relief of insomnia, stress reduction, and pain alleviation. But a 1989 report from the Centers for Disease Control connected tryptophan to a fatal blood disorder. As it happened, the problem was a contamination in the supply of a foreign manufacturer; however, the Food and Drug Administration (FDA) has continued to suspend the sale of over-the-counter tryptophan products.

As with other supplements, you should take tryptophan only under your physician's direction. But feel free to weight your diet more heavily toward tryptophan-high foods if you have sleep disturbances or other complaints that this amino acid may help to relieve.

Extra Scientific Information

- Concentrations of taurine (an amino acid) in the cerebrospinal fluid (clear fluid surrounding the brain and spinal cord) of patients with schizophrenia were 15 percent lower than in a group of healthy controls, according to 1995 research done at the Brain Research Institute, University of Zurich, Switzerland. *Note:* Taurine helps regulate

the nervous system and the muscles. (See *Journal of Neurochemistry*, December 1995, pp. 2652-62.)
- Taurine can protect the heart from injuries that result from "reperfusion injury" after a heart attack, according to 1995 research done at the Universitat Munchen, Germany. This type of injury typically begins during ischemia, when the heart is cut off from blood flow during surgery or a heart attack. The blood then rushes back into the starved tissue and causes damage through oxidative stress, with the release of destructive free radicals (unstable oxygen molecules). The researchers concluded that taurine provided protection as an antioxidant by neutralizing the free radicals. (See *Free Radical Biology and Medicine*, October 1995, pp. 461-71.)
- The availability of the essential amino acid tryptophan at certain times of the year has been linked in a 1995 Belgian study to a lower incidence of suicide and depression. (See *Archives of General Psychiatry*, November 1995, pp. 937-46.)
- Women with bulimia nervosa *and* with a depletion of their tryptophan levels were recently studied at the University of Pittsburgh School of Medicine. They exhibited an increase in caloric intake and mood irritability, primarily because of a deficiency of serotonin, which may be corrected by tryptophan. (See *American Journal of Psychiatry*, November 1995, pp. 1668-71.)
- Normal males were given amino acid mixtures designed to raise or lower tryptophan availability, and thus to raise or lower brain serotonin production, in a 1995 study at McGill University in Montreal. The researchers found that lowered tryptophan levels *plus* the ingestion of alcohol led to increased aggression. Their conclusion: Men with

low brain serotonin levels may be particularly susceptible to alcohol-induced violence. (See *Psychopharmacology*, June 1995, pp. 353-60.)

* Scientists at the University of Limburg, Maastricht,
the Netherlands, investigated whether taking extra
tryptophan into the brain (and thus producing more
of the relaxing serotonin) would cause greater
fatigue during exercise in trained athletes. The
study, which involved ten endurance-trained male
athletes, revealed that increasing or decreasing the
amount of tryptophan had no effect on exercise performance. (See *Journal of Physiology*, August 1,
1995, pp. 789-94.)

* Researchers at the University La Sapienza in Rome
concluded that low levels of tryptophan in the brain
could be associated with low serotonin activity in
autistic children. (See *Biomedical Pharmacotherapy*,
1995, pp. 288-92.)

Special Food Sources, Strategies, and Facts

Certain food sources are weighted relatively heavily
toward the four amino acids discussed in the "Basic
Nutritional Therapy" section above. But remember: When
excess amino acids are consumed, they are oxidized or converted to fat or glucose, rather than used for additional protein synthesis. There are no official recommendations
(RDAs) for amino acids, and it is advisable to take supplements only under a doctor's supervision.

* *Arginine sources:* oat flakes (fortified), cooked oatmeal, wheat germ (toasted), dairy products (especially cottage cheese, ricotta cheese, nonfat dry milk,
plain skim yogurt), beef (especially red meats,
including chuck roast, various steak cuts, but *not*
ground meat), pork (especially Canadian bacon,
ham, shoulder), nuts (especially almonds, Brazil

nuts, peanuts), seeds (especially pumpkin, sesame, sunflower), poultry (especially chicken light meat and leg, turkey light meat), wild game (pheasant, quail), seafood (especially halibut, lobster, salmon, shrimp, snails, tuna in water), green peas, cooked soybeans.

- *Lysine sources:* oat flakes (fortified), dairy foods (especially milk, cottage cheese, ricotta cheese, eggs, yogurt), beef (especially red meats, including chuck roast, flank steak, round steak, sirloin steak, T-bone steak, tenderloin steak, but *not* ground meat), pork (especially Canadian bacon, boneless ham, various cuts), nuts (especially peanuts, pistachios), seeds (especially pumpkin, sesame, sunflower), poultry (especially chicken dark meat, domesticated duck and goose, turkey light meat), wild game (pheasant, quail), seafood (especially tuna in water: one can provides one of the best sources of lysine for a relatively small quantity of food), cooked soybeans, yeast, potatoes, lima beans.

- *Phenylalanine sources:* toasted wheat germ, dairy products (especially cottage cheese, ricotta cheese, nonfat dry milk), beef (especially chuck roast, various steak cuts), pork (especially Canadian bacon, boneless ham, various cuts), nuts (especially almonds, peanuts, pistachios), seeds (especially pumpkin, sesame, sunflower), poultry (especially chicken dark meat, chicken breast, chicken leg, domesticated goose), wild game (pheasant, quail), seafood (especially pickled herring and tuna in water), soybeans, bananas, lima beans.

- *Tryptophan sources:* beef (especially red meats, including chuck roast, various steak cuts, *not* ground beef), pork (especially Canadian bacon, boneless ham, leg and shoulder cuts, loin chop), nuts (especially almonds and peanuts), seeds (especially pumpkin, sesame, sunflower), poultry (especially chicken breast and leg, domesticated duck, turkey light meat), canned tuna in water, dried dates, milk, cottage cheese, bananas.

Therapy Recommendations

Unless you are under specific instructions from your physician, get your amino acids and protein from foods, not from supplements. Still, if you have special concerns or health goals, feel free to weight your diet toward the specific foods that contain the amino acids most likely to move you toward your objectives.

For example, if you are involved in fairly heavy exercise, including both strength and endurance training, you may be interested in getting plenty of arginine for muscle building. This means that you might design your diet to include relatively large proportions of foods like wheat germ, cottage cheese, ricotta cheese, plain skim yogurt, chuck roast, various loin cuts of steak (*not* ground beef), peanuts, sesame and sunflower seeds, salmon, scallops, shrimp, canned tuna in water, green peas, and cooked soybeans.

On the other hand, if your goal is to stabilize your emotions and perhaps get more sleep, you may focus on tryptophan. As a result, in your daily food program you might emphasize a diet that overlaps with the one for arginine, but still has its distinctive features. This would include such foods as chuck roast, various loin steak cuts (*not* ground beef), boneless ham, almonds, peanuts, pumpkin seeds, sesame seeds, sunflower seeds, chicken breast and legs, domesticated duck, turkey (light meat), and canned tuna in water.

Of course, there is no guarantee that adjusting your diet in such ways will actually enable you to achieve your goals. But there is nutritional evidence that specific nutrients can make a difference. You have nothing to lose as long as you make sure that you continue to eat an overall balanced diet.

Cross-References

See "Protein," "Insomnia," "Meat," "Soybeans and Soy Products."

ANEMIAS

An anemia is a condition where the size or number of red blood cells (erythrocytes) is deficient, where the hemoglobin within those cells has decreased, or where both of these conditions exist. Anemias can be classified according to the size of the red blood cells or the amount of hemoglobin they contain. (Note: hemoglobin is the pigment in red blood cells that carries oxygen to the tissues.)

Nutritional factors that may contribute to anemias include deficiencies of vitamin B_{12}, folic acid, or iron. Other nutritional anemias result from dietary deficiencies of protein, vitamin B_6, ascorbic acid (vitamin C), copper, or other heavy metals. The deficiency can arise from inadequate food intake, inability to absorb food or utilize it, or injury to the bone marrow.

Also, the increased requirement for certain nutrients during pregnancy or adolescence may lead to anemias. In addition, blood loss, such as from a wound or injury, also may trigger a type of anemia.

Basic Nutritional Therapy

Pernicious anemia, a condition found primarily in people over age fifty, is caused by a deficiency of vitamin B_{12}. (See the discussion under the entry "Pernicious Anemia.") The treatment of pernicious anemia and some other nutritional anemias, such as various malabsorption syndromes, is to increase the intake of vitamin B_{12}, especially through injections.

With folic acid deficiencies, supplemental folic acid is the antidote. In cases of iron deficiency from blood loss, iron supplements (ferrous sulfate) are used. With disorders involving red blood cell development, vitamin B_6 (pyridoxine) is the treatment of choice.

Obviously, before you attempt any treatment, a physician should first make the correct diagnosis of the cause of the anemia and then prescribe the appropriate response.

Extra Scientific Information

Here are some other points and principles to keep in mind about anemias:

- Because of a lack of a good source of iron in their diets, vegetarians must pay particular attention to preventing iron deficiency anemias. Still, it is possible for vegetarians to obtain adequate iron intake from plant foods and supplemental iron, and thus to avoid nutritional anemia. For suggestions, see the "Iron" entry.

- Excessive physical activity can cause an anemia due to destruction of red blood cells. At times, this condition can be completely corrected with supplemental iron, or if necessary, with intravenous injections. Evaluating for the blood level of ferritin will occasionally reveal an iron deficiency, even if a person has what appears to be a normal blood count of red blood cells and hemoglobin. Iron supplements such as ferrous sulfate can correct a ferritin deficiency and may also improve athletic or physical performance.

Note: At one time it was felt that excessive levels of iron in the blood might be a factor in causing coronary heart disease. A low level of iron during menstruation was seen as the primary reason that premenopausal women had some protection from heart disease. But later studies have disproved this theory and have actually shown some protection from heart disease in people with elevated hemoglobin.

- Anemias similar to those that may occur with blood loss can be caused by a number of other chronic medical problems, such as hypothyroidism, adrenal insufficiency, kidney disease, and cirrhosis of the liver.

Special Food Sources, Strategies, and Facts

See discussions in the entries entitled "Vitamin B_6," "Vitamin B_{12}," "Iron," and in Chapters 2 and 3.

Therapy Recommendations

Low grade iron deficiency or nutritional anemias can usually be corrected by increasing the intake of foods high in iron or by taking iron supplements. More severe anemias may require intramuscular or intravenous injections of iron. But all anemias must be treated by a physician after a correct diagnosis. This is not a condition where you should try self-diagnosis or treatment.

Cross-References

See "Vitamin B_6," "Vitamin B_{12}," "Iron," and Chapters 2 and 3.

ASPIRIN

It may seem strange to include aspirin in a book on nutrition, but this over-the-counter medication is so widely taken as a supplement that some comments are necessary.

First of all, a few facts: Aspirin, the common name for

acetylsalicylic acid, has been designated medically as a "nonsteroidal anti-inflammatory drug" (NSAID). It has long been used as an antidote to a variety of specific symptoms and health conditions, such as:

- Relieving various bodily pains, including head-aches, backaches, and arthritis discomfort
- Lowering fever
- Reducing inflammation

In more recent years, scientific studies have prompted many people, including many physicians, to begin taking regular doses as a preventive measure against heart disease, stroke, and cancer.

But despite this prevalent use, *not everyone* should take aspirin, as is evident in the following discussion.

Basic Nutritional Therapy

Aspirin may be taken safely by most healthy adults for pain relief, fever management, and reduction of inflammation accompanying a condition like arthritis. (See "Warning!") But these common uses only scratch the surface of the possibilities for this wonder drug.

How about heart disease, stroke, and cancer? Recent studies have shown that aspirin can help to prevent heart attacks. The *British Medical Journal* reported in 1988 that there was a 30 percent decrease in stroke and heart attacks among 29,000 heart and stroke patients who took one 325-milligram aspirin tablet daily.

In another study published in the same year in the *New England Journal of Medicine,* more than 10,000 physicians with no history of heart problems took one aspirin tablet (325 milligrams) every other day. After five years, the doctors on the aspirin had half the rate of heart attacks of a control group of doctors who did not take aspirin.

In a 1995 article in the *New England Journal of*

Medicine, medical researchers concluded that taking four to six aspirin tablets a week could substantially reduce the risk of women for cancer of the colon. But the greatest reduction in cancer resulted in those women who took the aspirin regularly for at least twenty years.

Warning!

Aspirin should be avoided for any of the above purposes if you have the following health problems: a bleeding disorder (aspirin can promote bleeding); stomach irritations or related problems such as ulcers, gout, liver disease, or asthma. Bleeding inside the head rarely occurs in people who take aspirin as a preventive measure.

Other important warnings: Pregnant and breast-feeding women may need to avoid the drug because it may pose a danger to their unborn child or infant. Also, because of the possibility of developing Reye's syndrome (a rare childhood disease that may result in high fever, coma, and death), teenagers and younger children should avoid aspirin if they are suffering from a viral illness, flu, or chicken pox. Finally, patients taking an anticoagulant drug such as Coumadin should restrict usage of this medication.

In any case, always check with your doctor before you use aspirin on a regular basis, particularly before going on aspirin as a preventive measure against cardiovascular disease or cancer. Some doctors feel that despite the studies showing the decrease in risk, regular ingestion of aspirin should be reserved only for those patients who already have diagnosed heart disease or have multiple coronary risk factors. A strong history of colon cancer is another possible reason to use aspirin "prophylactically," or as a preventive measure. Your physician is in the best position to advise you as to whether you are a candidate for this therapy.

Extra Scientific Information

• In a September 7, 1995, article in the *New England Journal of Medicine*, medical researchers at Harvard reported that the cancer-protective effects of an aspirin tablet every other day began to show up only after ten years, with the maximum benefits occurring after twenty years.

In an accompanying editorial, Dr. Aaron J. Marcus of the Veterans Affairs Medical Center in New York said he would recommend that people at risk for colorectal cancer—and also those with inflammatory bowel disease, cancers of the breast, ovaries, or large bowels—should take a single aspirin tablet every other day. Also, those with a family history of colon cancer should do the same. But those with aspirin-related medical risks or conditions should avoid the drug. (See the *New England Journal of Medicine*, September 7, 1995, pp. 609-14.)

• The average American takes in the equivalent of one baby aspirin a day (80 milligrams) from foods that are artificially flavored, according to a report by researchers from the National Center for Health Statistics in Hyattsville, Maryland. This finding was presented at a March 1996 conference in San Francisco of the American Heart Association.

The artificially flavored foods contain salicylate, a chemical cousin of aspirin. Researchers said this fact may partly explain why deaths from heart attacks have declined over the last thirty years. Of course, other important reasons for this decline include more exercise, less smoking, lower intake of saturated fats, and better medical care.

Special Food Sources, Strategies, and Facts

In most of the studies conducted on aspirin, the standard dose given is the 325 milligram tablet taken every other day. Some physicians have suggested that an 80 milligram children's tablet taken daily will do just as well, and that may be true. But at this point, the research is not solid.

As for the type of aspirin tablet, most physicians feel that the coated variety, which will not dissolve in the stomach, is safest for preventing irritation of the lining of the stomach and stomach ulcers.

Therapy Recommendations

If you are *not* in any of the groups listed under the "Warning!" section above, taking a 325-milligram aspirin every other day or a baby aspirin daily shouldn't hurt, and might very well help to prevent heart disease and colon cancer. But there is a slight increase in the risk of intracranial (inside the skull) bleeding.

If you *are* in a high-risk group for heart disease, stroke, or colon cancer, you should seriously consider aspirin as a preventive measure. But if you do go on this regimen, be sure to first get the approval of your physician.

Cross-References

See "Asthma," "Cancers," "Heart Disease."

ASTHMA

Asthma attacks may be prompted by a variety of factors, including: excessive exercise, cold weather, stress, or allergic reactions to such substances as drugs (e.g., aspirin), pollen, dust, or animal hair. But a commonly overlooked trigger for asthma can be certain foods. *Note:* Children are particularly vulnerable to food triggers for asthma.

Basic Nutritional Therapy

Some children with asthma, who are also allergic to at least one food, may fail to respond positively to asthma treatment unless they avoid the offending food, according to researchers from Johns Hopkins Children's Center in Baltimore.

This American Lung Association study, published in the February 1996 issue of the *American Journal of Respiratory and Critical Care Medicine*, involved twenty-six children with food allergies. Each child was given a food known to cause an allergic reaction in that child.

Twelve of the children developed asthma-like respiratory symptoms, such as coughing, wheezing, or a tight feeling in the chest. Seven of those twelve suffered from irritable airways or related symptoms that are common precursors to an asthma attack. The foods producing these symptoms included eggs, wheat, cow's milk, soy, and fish.

The researchers concluded that children with hard-to-manage asthma should be checked for food allergies through food elimination or skin testing.

Special Food Sources, Strategies, and Facts

Foods to watch if you or a family member has asthma: eggs, wheat, cow's milk, soy, and fish. (Since this is not an exhaustive list, your physician should help you identify other foods that may produce allergic reactions.)

Therapy Recommendations

Any testing for food allergies should be conducted by a physician who is a qualified allergy specialist. Usually, the specialist will place the patient on a restricted diet and then introduce a variety of foods, one at a time, until an allergic or asthmatic reaction occurs. When the offending food has been identified, it can be eliminated from the patient's diet.

Cross-References

See "Allergies and Food Intolerances," "Asprin."

ATHEROSCLEROSIS, ARTERIOSCLEROSIS

Poor nutrition is only one of many factors that may contribute to the development of atherosclerosis, which is the hardening or clogging of the inner lining (intima) of the arteries with lipid (fatty) deposits and plaque. This condition, which may eventually shut off the blood flow to the heart or brain, is the primary culprit in most heart attacks and strokes. The more general term, *arteriosclerosis*, may also be used for this disease.

Your genetic background is a strong risk factor. If one of your parents died of a cardiovascular disease, especially before age fifty, your own risk increases significantly. Also, you will face greater dangers of developing atherosclerosis if certain other characteristics are present in your life: a sedentary lifestyle, a failure to handle stress well, a naturally high or unbalanced cholesterol profile, cigarette smoking, or high blood pressure.

Some of these conditions are not within your power to change. However, there is one very powerful risk factor that you *can* control: a poorly managed diet.

Basic Nutritional Therapy

The space limits of this section prevent me from providing a complete explanation of how good nutrition and a wise use of supplements can help lower your risk of atherosclerosis. For more detailed treatment of this subject, you should consult my other books, especially *Antioxidant Revolution* (Thomas Nelson, 1994), *Controlling Cholesterol* (Bantam, 1988), and *The Aerobics Program for Total Well-Being* (Bantam, 1982).

What I can do here is to give you an overview, which you can use as a checklist to see if your nutritional program is on track. Here are the main points:

- Keep your daily intake of fats below 30 percent of your total daily consumption of calories. (See "Fat.")

The reason for this rule: A high intake of fats, especially saturated fats, will contribute to the manufacture of cholesterol in your blood. An excess of cholesterol will increase your risk of developing the fatty deposits in your arteries that lead to atherosclerosis.

Assuming that you consume a total of 2,400 calories a day, you should be taking in no more than 720 (30 percent) of those calories as fat.

To figure this out, you will first have to find the number of grams of fat in your food. This information is available from nutritional labels on the food you buy or in nutritional charts such as those I have included in the books listed above.

Next, you have to know that 1 gram of fat produces 9 calories. So the maximum number of grams of fat you should take in daily would be 80 (720 calories divided by 9 calories per gram = 80 grams).

- Be sure that your intake of *saturated* fats, such as butter, much of the fat in whole milk and whole milk cheese, or the visible fat on beef or other meats, is limited to no more than one-third of your fat calories per day, or about 10 percent of your total calories. (See "Fat.")
- Emphasize *monounsaturated fats*, such as olive oil, in your diet rather than saturated fats. This type of fat, consumed in large quantities, has been associated with a lower incidence of atherosclerosis, especially in countries along the Mediterranean. (See "Fat.")
- Take 400 to 800 micrograms of folic acid per day.

There is evidence that this therapy will lower the level of homocysteines in your blood. High blood levels of these components of protein are increasingly regarded as a risk factor for cardiovascular disease. (See "Folic Acid, Folate," and also the discussion in Part I of this book.)

- Take at least 400 IUs (international units) of natural vitamin E every day (supplements of d-alpha tocopherol).

This nutrient, which cannot easily be consumed in sufficient quantities solely through the diet, has been linked in various studies to a lower incidence of cardiovascular disease. It is believed to fight the destructive action of free radicals in the body, which can cause oxidation of the low-density lipoprotein (LDL) component of cholesterol. This oxidation furthers the process of atherosclerosis by promoting the formation of plaque on artery walls. (See "Vitamin E," and the discussions on antioxidants in Part I of this book.)

- Take in at least 500 to 1,000 milligrams of vitamin C every day. Because it's hard to take in this much vitamin C every day through the diet, I recommend that most people rely on supplements as well. But you should still emphasize vitamin C-rich foods in your diet, such as strawberries, orange juice, and cranberry juice cocktail. (For a detailed list of such foods, see my *Antioxidant Revolution*, p. 150.)

One reason vitamin C is so important is that, like vitamin E, it has been linked to a lower incidence of cardiovascular disease. In particular, vitamin C is regarded as a kind of "helper" that enhances the beneficial effect of vitamin E. (See "Vitamin C," and also the discussion on antioxidants in Part I.)

- Eat foods high in beta-carotene. It's best to get beta-carotene through your diet, and that is fairly easy. For example, to take in 25,000 IUs a day, the minimum requirement for the greatest health benefits, you only need to eat one large carrot or one baked sweet potato.

Supplements are also an option, but probably should be avoided by smokers or heavy drinkers because of possible health complications. (See "Vitamin A" and also the discussion of antioxidants in Part I.)

- Include plenty of foods with soluble fiber in your diet, such as oat bran, oatmeal, lentils, and dried beans.

The reason for these selections is that a number of studies have indicated that soluble fiber helps to "mop up" excess cholesterol in your small intestines. (See "Cholesterol," "Fiber, Soluble.")

- Lose weight. Obesity is usually related to higher total cholesterol levels and lower HDLs. The less you weigh, the lower your total cholesterol and the higher your HDLs tend to be. (See "Obesity.")

Therapy Recommendations

My basic dietary and food supplement recommendations to prevent atherosclerosis have been incorporated in the above section on "Basic Nutritional Therapy."

Cross-References

See "Vitamin A," "Cholesterol," "Vitamin E," "Fat," "Mediterranean Diet," "Obesity." Also, consult Part I, which contains the latest information on antioxidants.

B VITAMINS

VITAMIN B₁ (THIAMINE)

Vitamin B_1, also known as thiamine, is necessary for a number of bodily operations. These include maintaining the nervous system, helping the metabolism of carbohydrates, overall growth, and skin health.

Those with a serious vitamin B_1 deficiency may also develop beriberi. This disease can cause general weakness, fatigue, calf muscle pain, upset stomach, constipation, neuritis (inflammation and degeneration of the nerves), and sometimes even mental problems, such as irritability and depression. It can also be a factor in heart failure. Alcoholics and those who eat a diet mainly of unenriched white rice or white flour products are particularly susceptible to vitamin B_1-related problems.

Basic Nutritional Therapy

The Recommended Dietary Allowance (RDA) for vitamin B_1 is 1.5 milligrams per day for men up to fifty years of age, and 1.2 mg for men over fifty. The RDA for women up to age fifty is 1.1 mg daily, and 1.0 mg for women over fifty. Although much larger amounts are taken by many people without negative results, it's better to get vitamin B_1 through food rather than through a supplement. (See "Food Sources.")

Megadoses (up to about 50 milligrams a day or even more) may very well benefit heavy drinkers, those with a poor diet and appetite (especially the elderly), and patients with any of the symptoms mentioned above. In fact, many physicians prescribe thiamine for alcoholics, especially those suffering from Wernicke's Syndrome. This condition is characterized by dangerously low blood pressure and a paralysis of muscles controlling lateral eye movements. Intravenous thiamine can temporarily restore eye muscle function, but unfortunately this is usually a terminal condition.

Extra Scientific Information

- In a 1995 study, a significant proportion of patients with Alzheimer's disease had a thiamine deficiency, and this may have had an impact on their mental functioning, according to researchers from the Department of Neurology, University of South Florida College of Medicine in Tampa. (See the November 1995 issue of *Archives of Neurology*, pp. 1081-6.)

- In a 1995 investigation, twenty-seven inmates from a Malaysian detention center were evaluated for possible causes of ankle swelling. Three of the patients were suffering from heart failure, and 40 percent had other heart abnormalities. The researchers found that all of the patients showed a prompt, positive clinical response to thiamine replacement therapy, according to the *Medical Journal of Malaysia*, March 1995, pp. 17-20.

- Large oral thiamine supplements (200 milligrams taken daily for six weeks) resulted in improvement of the function of the left ventricle of the heart in a group of patients with congestive heart failure. Researchers from the Division of Clinical Pharmacology, Sheba Medical Center, Tel-Hashomer, Israel, concluded that patients with moderate to severe heart failure should consider such thiamine therapy.

Special Food Sources, Strategies, and Facts

Good food sources for vitamin B_1 (thiamine) include the following: fortified wheat flakes, toasted wheat germ, brewer's yeast, raw peanuts, rice bran, millet, lamb, Canadian bacon, ham, various pork cuts, venison, quail, black beans (especially dried beans), green peas, sunflower seeds, and watermelon.

Therapy Recommendations

If you are a heavy drinker or know that your diet is unbalanced or your appetite is low, perhaps because of advanced age, you should emphasize thiamine-rich foods in your diet. Also, see your physician about the advisability of getting thiamine injections or taking megadoses of this vitamin. Caution: heavy drinkers still run the risk of a thiamine deficiency, even on megadoses of the vitamin. The best treatment is to decrease the alcohol intake to less than two drinks per day (a maximum of ten per week), or preferably, to abstain.

Cross-References

See "Alcohol," "Heart Disease."

VITAMIN B$_2$ (RIBOFLAVIN)

Vitamin B$_2$ (riboflavin) is important for the maintenance of healthy, supple skin; for good vision (possibly including the prevention or treatment of cataracts); and perhaps for the proper metabolism of glucose and fatty acids. This vitamin may also help relieve damage done to the body by excessive stress or exercise.

Signs of a riboflavin deficiency include sensitivity of the eyes to light, eye irritation, cracks in the lips (especially at the corners of the mouth), dry or scaly skin, carpal tunnel syndrome, and swelling in the legs.

Basic Nutritional Therapy

The RDA for vitamin B$_2$ is 1.7 milligrams daily for the average adult man, and 1.3 milligrams for the average adult woman. Dietitians recommend an extra .3 milligram for pregnant women and an extra .5 milligram for nursing women.

Some enthusiasts have recommended that the daily intake of this vitamin be upped to as much as 100 to 500 milligrams for treatment of stress, depression, cataracts, and a variety of other ills. However, I would advise that you avoid supplements unless your physician prescribes them. Instead, stick to riboflavin-high foods. (See "Food Sources.")

Extra Scientific Information

* When vitamin B_2 was administered to holstein cattle through intramuscular injection, there was a significant increase in their neutrophils, or white blood cells, according to researchers from Obihiro University in Hokkaido, Japan. (See *Journal of Veterinary Medicine and Science*, June 1995, pp. 493-5.)
* Researchers at the University of Michigan Medical School found that riboflavin supplements had a protective effect on animal hearts during reoxygenation, which involved first starving the heart of blood and then putting blood back into the organ. (See *Biochemical and Biophysical Research*, July 6, 1995, pp. 35-40.)
* Four patients studied at Erasmus University, Rotterdam, the Netherlands, had shown exercise intolerance since early childhood. But they developed greatly increased endurance, demonstrated through clinical exercise testing, as a result of taking high doses of riboflavin supplements. (See *Biochemical and Biophysical Acta*, May 24, 1995, pp. 75-83.)

Special Food Sources, Strategies, and Facts

Foods high in vitamin B_2 (riboflavin) include: fortified wheat flakes, toasted wheat germ, wild rice, brewer's yeast, milk (especially nonfat dry), yogurt, ricotta cheese, chuck roast, kidney, heart, dried eggs, spinach, oysters, many baby food cereals, liver, liverwurst, braunschweiger sausage, loin of lamb, dried chili powder (with seasoning), leg of pork, veal, venison, almonds, quail.

Therapy Recommendations

As you look over the preceding list of foods, you can immediately see that a number of them would be highly inappropriate for anyone remotely concerned about a heart-healthy, low-cholesterol diet. Despite the fact that organ meats like liver and heart are high in riboflavin, this benefit is outweighed by their high levels of cholesterol.

Some of the other choices, including the wheat flakes and toasted wheat germ cereals, wild rice, nonfat dry milk, venison, or lean steak cuts, might fit quite well into a cholesterol-restricted diet.

Most people who stick to riboflavin-rich foods will get plenty of this vitamin. But there is scientific authority that higher doses through supplementation may be in order for those dealing with such conditions as excessive fatigue or cataracts. If your physician feels you might benefit from extra B_2 through supplements, by all means try it.

Cross-References

See "Vitamin B_2," "Eye Complaints."

VITAMIN B_3 (NIACIN, NICOTINIC ACID)

Niacin, which is available under the name nicotinic acid, is important in promoting a healthy nervous system, skin, and gastrointestinal functioning. You can usually get all you need through foods rich in B_3. (See "Food Sources.")

In recent years, other important functions of niacin have become evident through many scientific studies. These include the lowering of total cholesterol in the blood and also the improved balancing of the subcomponents of cholesterol. For this type of therapy, however, megadoses of niacin are required, and *the approval of a qualified physician is absolutely essential!*

Basic Nutritional Therapy

The RDA for daily niacin intake for adults is 15 to 20 milligrams per day. Nonpregnant, nonlactating women should consume niacin in the lower part of that range; and men, pregnant women, and lactating women in the upper range. (See "Food Sources.")

Those who are deficient in dietary niacin may experience a variety of health problems, including pellagra, a disease common among alcoholics, which includes body rashes, inflammation of the mouth and tongue, and mental deterioration. Those who regularly consume niacin-rich foods, such as fortified wheat flakes, bran flakes, various types of beef steaks, or toasted wheat germ—should have no problem with a niacin deficiency.

Is niacin a cholesterol wonder drug? Niacin is not a wonder drug; but used properly in relatively large doses, it can provide tremendous benefits for many people with cholesterol problems, particularly low levels of "good" HDLs. For the details on this therapy, please refer to my *Controlling Cholesterol* (Bantam Paperback, 1989). In a nutshell, here is the basic approach:

• First, do not try to use megadoses of niacin on your own to control a cholesterol problem. Because of the possibly serious side effects of this drug (yes, it *is* a drug when used in large amounts), it is absolutely essential that you proceed only under a doctor's direction.

One of the most serious side effects is liver damage in some people who take megadoses (as little as 500 milligrams daily). As a result, it's important for those on large amounts of niacin to have regular blood tests to monitor their liver functions.

- Generally speaking, niacin as a cholesterol-control medication is recommended in doses of about 1,500 to 3,000 milligrams per day.
- Regular, nontimed-release tablets should be used. Timed-release (or sustained-release) tablets have been linked to a higher incidence of liver problems and other negative side effects.
- Expect some flushing or the development of a temporary rash when you first go on the higher doses. This side effect should disappear as your body becomes used to the medication. The flushing can be minimized by taking the tablets in several smaller doses over the course of the day, preferably during meals, or by taking an aspirin tablet with the niacin.

Many people on this type of niacin therapy have found that their total cholesterol drops significantly, by 20 percent or more. Also, the decrease tends to be in their "bad" cholesterol (the LDL, or low-density lipoprotein, which has been associated with a higher risk of cardiovascular disease). Furthermore, niacin often causes the "good" cholesterol (HDL, or high-density lipoprotein, which is linked to protection against heart disease) to stay steady or even rise. When used with other cholesterol-lowering medications, the results can be even more dramatic. (See "Extra Scientific Information.") It's no wonder that many people regard niacin as something of a wonder drug!

Extra Scientific Information

- Nicotinic acid (niacin) in both regular and sustained-release forms is a powerful drug when used in high doses (1,000 milligrams or more) to treat lipid disorders such as high cholesterol, according to an

October 1995 article in the *American Journal of Medicine* (pp. 378-85). The researchers, from our Cooper Clinic in Dallas, also confirmed that niacin may cause disturbing side effects such as liver problems, especially when it is employed on a long-term basis. As a result, the drug should be used only under the continuing, careful supervision of a physician.

- Investigators from the Gatorade Sports Science Institute in Barrington, Illinois, reported in the July 1995 issue of *Medical Science Sports and Exercise* (pp. 1057-62) that using niacin to blunt the normal rise of free fatty acids alters the hormonal response to exercise and reduces the person's capacity to perform high-intensity exercise.

- Niacin may be the most cost-effective lipid-lowering agent currently available, the journal *Postgraduate Medicine* reported in August 1995 (pp. 185-9, 192-3).

- A combination of nicotinic acid and the drug Pravastatin is more effective than Pravastatin alone in reducing levels of triglycerides and elevating "good" HDL cholesterol, and lowering total cholesterol, according to the *Journal of Cardiovascular Risk,* October 1994 (pp. 231-9). Also, the combination is more effective than nicotinic acid alone in reducing total cholesterol, triglycerides, and "bad" LDL cholesterol.

- The combination of nicotinic acid (1,200 milligrams per day) and lovastatin or mevacor (20 milligrams per day) is more effective than either drug alone in reducing total and "bad" LDL cholesterol, the *American Journal of Cardiology* reported in its July 15, 1995, issue (pp. 182-4).

- A sixty-one-year-old white man with high cholesterol levels developed pruritus (itching) and jaundice (yellowish coloring in the skin) after taking 3 grams of nicotinic acid daily for thirteen months. Researchers at the Lutheran Medical Center in Cleveland concluded in the January-February 1994 *Cleveland Clinic Journal of Medicine* that jaundice induced by nicotinic acid may be more common than previously thought. Physicians should be alert to this symptom in patients taking the drug (pp. 70-5, 80-2).

• The sustained-release form of niacin is toxic to the liver and should be restricted from use, scientists at the School of Pharmacy, Medical College of Virginia concluded in the *Journal of the American Medical Association* (March 2, 1994, pp. 672-7). Furthermore, though the immediate-release variety of niacin is to be preferred in treating high cholesterol, it can also cause significant adverse effects. Consequently, niacin supplements should be given only to patients who can be monitored carefully by experienced health professionals.

• Scientists at the University of Southern California School of Medicine in Los Angeles found an association between reduction in progression of clogging of the coronary arteries and the intake of at least 100 IUs of vitamin E *plus* a niacin-colestipol drug combination. (See *Journal of the American Medical Association*, June 21, 1995, pp. 1849-54.)

• In a study in rural China, persons receiving a combination of riboflavin and niacin experienced a significantly lower prevalence of age-related cataracts. (See *Archives of Ophthalmology*, September 1993, pp. 1246-53.)

Special Food Sources, Strategies, and Facts

Although the megadoses of niacin needed to affect cholesterol levels must be obtained from supplements, a number of foods contain plenty of this vitamin for the average person's needs. These include: bagels, wheat, fortified wheat bran flakes, toasted wheat germ, wheat bran, rice bran, brown rice, wild rice, mushrooms, baked potatoes, chuck roast, various beef steak cuts, beef liver, lamb, pork, veal, wild game, peanuts, sesame seeds, chicken breast, duck, goose, turkey (light meat), tuna, halibut, swordfish, and brewer's yeast.

Therapy Recommendations

Unless you have a problem with your blood lipids (such as high cholesterol), stick to dietary sources for your niacin.

If you have a cholesterol or other type of lipid problem, your physician may recommend niacin as a means of treatment. *But don't try to treat yourself!* Niacin is an easily obtained, inexpensive, over-the-counter medication that can be quite tempting to use for self-treatment. But as you have seen in the above scientific findings, this vitamin is also a powerful drug that can cause serious harm if it is used without proper supervision.

Cross-References

See "Heart Disease," "Atherosclerosis."

VITAMIN B₆ (PYRIDOXINE)

Vitamin B_6 (pyridoxine), which is present in small to moderate amounts in many of our foods (see "Food Sources" below), plays a role in several enzyme-related tasks in the body's protein metabolism and cell function.

A deficiency, more of a problem for infants than adults, may cause skin irritations, convulsions, anemia, and retarded growth. When used in relatively large doses, this nutrient has been linked to a number of possible health benefits.

Basic Nutritional Therapy

The possible uses of B_6 in nutritional therapy include:

- Some relief of carpal tunnel syndrome, a condition triggered by overuse of wrist muscles and ligaments through activities such as excessive typing, resulting in pain and weakness in the wrist area. Physicians using this experimental treatment have sometimes recommended taking B_6 with riboflavin (vitamin B_2).
- Relief of premenstrual syndrome symptoms in many women.
- Relief of depression.
- Relief of some convulsions and seizures in infants, including those suffering from epilepsy.
- Relief of some symptoms of asthma, including wheezing.
- Relief of nausea and vomiting during pregnancy. (See "Extra Scientific Information.")

Extra Scientific Information

Pyridoxine is effective in relieving the severity of nausea in early pregnancy, according to researchers at the Faculty of Medicine, Chiang Mai University, Thailand. During an eleven-month period, they monitored 342 women, who had been pregnant for seventeen weeks at the beginning of the study. Half of the participants received 30 milligrams a day of pyridoxine hydrochloride and the other half a placebo.

The result: There was a significant decrease in nausea in those women taking pyridoxine. (See *American Journal of Obstetrics and Gynecology*, September 1995, pp. 881-4.)

Special Food Sources, Strategies, and Facts

Although the RDA for pyridoxine is only about 2 milligrams per day, higher amounts up to about 100 milligrams per day are safe for most people. But because of possible side effects, you should take B_6 supplements *only* under the guidance of a physician.

Warning: When a person begins to take more than about 100 milligrams, symptoms such as tingling or numbness in the extremities may occur. Very high doses, in the range of 2 to 3 grams (2,000 to 3,000 milligrams), may produce more severe symptoms, such as temporary inability to walk.

Also, this vitamin should be avoided by patients taking the drug levodopa, which is used to treat Parkinson's disease.

Because of the possibility of overdosing through supplements, I generally recommend that most people stick to getting their pyridoxine through their diet, unless a personal physician directs otherwise.

Foods with relatively high amounts of vitamin B_6 include: fortified bran oat and wheat flakes, toasted wheat germ, soy flour, wheat bran, baked potatoes, avocados, bananas, dried figs, chuck roast, various beef steak cuts (*not* ground beef), beef livers, lamb, pork, veal, wild game, fresh chestnuts, hazelnuts, peanuts, sunflower seeds, walnuts, chicken (especially light meat), duck, goose, turkey (light meat), salmon, trout, carrot juice, tomato paste, brewer's yeast, watermelon, spinach.

Therapy Recommendations

Most people should get their vitamin B_6 from foods.

Those with special problems—such as severe premenstrual syndrome, carpal tunnel syndrome, depression, or infants with convulsion-type problems—may be candidates for supplements. For example, certain gynecologists will prescribe high doses of B_6 to patients who suffer from PMS; a daily dose of 300 milligrams is common.

Caution: Do *not* go on pyridoxine supplements, especially in higher doses of 100 milligrams or more, without checking first with your doctor.

Cross-References

See "Vitamin B_2," "Carpal Tunnel Syndrome," Chapter 3.

VITAMIN B_{12} (COBALAMIN)

Vitamin B_{12} plays a major role in the metabolism of protein, fats, and sugars, including the absorption and conversion of folate (folic acid) into its active form. B_{12} is also important in fostering the process of growth, and for helping the body to form blood. One of the most important functions of this vitamin is to help maintain the sheath (myelin) that develops around each of the body's nerves. When this nerve sheath falls into disrepair, nervous disorders may result.

A deficiency in this vitamin may result in pernicious anemia or neuritis (inflammation or degeneration of a nerve). Relatively high doses of folic acid may mask the symptoms of pernicious anemia. As a result, everyone taking more than 1,000 micrograms of folic acid per day, and also anyone on folic acid who is over fifty, should be taking vitamin B_{12} supplements. (See "Therapy Recommendations" and also the discussion in Chapter 3.)

Note: Because Vitamin B_{12} is found largely in animal products, vegetarians have to be careful to consume plenty of milk, cheese, and eggs to supplement their diets adequately. (See "Food Sources." Note that ample amounts of vitamin B_{12} can also be found in some wheat foods and fortified cereals.)

Basic Nutritional Therapy

The RDA for vitamin B_{12} is only 2 *micro*grams per day (be sure to distinguish this amount from *milli*grams: a microgram is one-millionth of a gram, while a milligram is one-thousandth of a gram). Those with pernicious anemia may be required by their doctors to have B_{12} injections (*not* oral supplements).

Pernicious anemia involves the lack of a protein-related compound called the "intrinsic factor." This factor is required for the body to absorb B_{12}. A B_{12} deficiency may result in numbness in the body, a stumbling walk, early signs of senility, or unusual fatigue.

Extra Scientific Information

- Adherents to a strict, uncooked "vegan" diet—one permitting no animal food *or* dairy products, also called the "living food diet"—were evaluated as to their vitamin B_{12} status by nutritional researchers at the University of Kuopio, Finland (see *Journal of Nutrition*, October 1995, pp. 2511-5).

The researchers found that the vegans had a significantly lower blood level of B_{12} than participants on a non-vegetarian diet. (But the vegans who consumed significant amounts of Nori and Chlorella seaweeds had blood serum levels of B_{12} twice as high as the vegans not using those seaweeds, though they were still lower than the levels of the nonvegetarians.)

This topic is highly controversial since vitamin B_{12} is found almost exclusively in animal flesh and animal products. The amounts of vitamin B_{12} listed on labels of plant products are inaccurate because the B_{12} in these products occurs in inactive, unavailable form.

- Researchers at the Department of Psychophysiology, National Institute of Mental Health, Ichikawa, Japan studied the effect of vitamin B_{12} on the human circadian clock, the daylong human biological cycle or "inner clock." They found that intravenous injection of a form of B_{12} increased the rectal temperature during later daytime hours. As a result, alertness of the participants increased.

The investigators concluded that vitamin B_{12} may have a significant effect on the circadian clock. (See *Neuroscience Letters*, June 1995, pp. 1-4.)

- Severely disturbed wake-sleep rhythms may be improved by the administration of vitamin B_{12}, according to an August 18, 1995, report in the journal *Life Sciences* (pp. 1317-23).

Special Food Sources, Strategies, and Facts

The best food sources of vitamin B_{12} are: fortified bran, oat and wheat flakes, toasted wheat germ, skim milk, whole milk, nonfat dry milk, ricotta cheese, creamed cottage cheese, dry cottage cheese, lowfat cottage cheese, plain low-fat and skim yogurt, chuck roast and various beef steak cuts (a very rich source!), lamb, pork, veal, chicken and turkey liver, and most fish—especially bass, bluefish, crab, herring, mackerel, salmon, snails, trout.

Therapy Recommendations

For those suffering from pernicious anemia, intravenous injections are necessary to get the benefits of B_{12} supplementation.

Those without pernicious anemia who are taking large doses of folic acid (1,000 micrograms per day or more), or who are over fifty years of age, should take B_{12} supplements daily. A good rule of thumb is to take 200 mcg of B_{12} for every 1,000 mcg of folic acid. (See Chapter 3.)

You can increase the amounts of B_{12} absorbed into your body (or "bioavailable") by getting this nutrient in larger doses through your diet. (See "Food Sources" to increase your dietary intake of B_{12} well above the RDA of 2 micrograms.)

Cross-References

See "Pernicious Anemia," and the discussions in Chapters 2 and 3.

BIOFLAVONOIDS

Bioflavonoids (Hesperidin and Rutin), also known as "vitamin P," are plant derivatives found in abundance in the white matter inside the peel of citrus fruits. These nutrients contain what is known as the "capillary permeability factor," which reduces the permeability and fragility of capillaries (tiny blood vessels, such as those feeding the skin). The capillary permeability factor also plays a role in treating purpura (a discoloration resulting from hemorrhaging in the skin). There are indications that bioflavonoids may have a number of other health benefits. (See "Basic Nutritional Therapy.")

Basic Nutritional Therapy

As indicated above, bioflavonoids are useful in treating certain types of purpura. Furthermore, animal and limited human studies suggest they *may* help with these conditions:

- Increasing the bioavailability of vitamin C.
- Possible anticarcinogenic activity (protection from cancer) through antioxidant action as scavengers of free radicals. (See "Extra Scientific Information.")

- Reducing cholesterol levels in some patients.
- Prevention of cataracts.

Extra Scientific Information

A number of recent scientific studies have shown these possibilities for bioflavonoids and their derivatives:

- Flavonoids, such as those found in vegetables, fruits, tea, and wine are excellent scavengers of free radicals, which increasing numbers of experts believe are at least partially responsible for our high incidence of cancer and heart disease. In particular, Dutch researchers have concluded that flavonoids are successful in scavenging or neutralizing the destructive nitric oxide radical. (See *Biochemical and Biophysical Research*, September 25, 1995, pp. 755-59.)
- Dutch researchers measured the levels of five major flavonoids: quercetin, daempferol, myricetin, apigenin, and luteolin, in twenty-eight vegetables, twelve fruits, and nine beverages. The major sources of the flavonoids in the Dutch diet were black tea, onions, and apples.

Based on interviews by dietitians with 805 men, the researchers first estimated the flavonoid intake in 1985. Five years later, they determined that forty-three men had died from heart disease. The researchers found that those who had consumed the most flavonoids had a 68 percent lower risk of dying than those who had consumed the least. This result may have occurred because "these flavonoids reduced the level of oxidized ["bad"] LDL cholesterol, thus inhibiting the growth of atherosclerotic plaques." (See *Lancet*, 1993, 324:1007.)

- Baicalin, a flavonoid compound, can protect the body's membranes from free radical injuries. Furthermore, this nutrient is even more effective when used with vitamin E. (See *Biochemistry and Molecular Biology International*, April 1995, pp. 981-94.)
- Baicalin may serve as a useful drug for the treatment of HIV infections, according to scientists at the National Cancer Institute-Frederick Cancer Research and Development Center in Maryland. (See *Cellular and Molecular Biology Research*, 1993, pp. 119-24.)
- Animal studies at the Faculty of Pharmaceutical Sciences, University of Jos, Nigeria, revealed that the leaves of the Baphia nitida plant, which is rich in flavonoids, can be used as an anti-inflammatory agent. (See *Journal of Ethnopharmacology*, May 1995, pp. 121-4.)
- A flavonoid derivative was used successfully to reduce bleeding that occurred after the removal of hemorrhoids. (See *British Journal of Surgery*, August 1995, pp. 1034-5.)

Special Food Sources, Strategies, and Facts

Good sources of bioflavonoids include: vegetables, the white matter inside the peel of oranges, grapefruits, and other citrus fruits, buckwheat, black currants, tea, and wine.

When you have a choice, take the whole citrus fruit, rather than the juice. Also, when you peel oranges, grapefruits, or other citrus fruits, be careful not to remove all the white matter just under the peel. In the past, you may have felt that this substance made the fruit too "chewy," but when you eliminate it, you are also eliminating important bioflavonoids.

Therapy Recommendations

Because the impact of megadoses of bioflavonoids on the human body is generally unknown, I recommend sticking to natural sources, such as those mentioned above. Large amounts of bioflavonoid supplements can cause diarrhea.

Cross-References

See "Vitamin C."

BIOTIN

Biotin, a component of the vitamin B_2 complex, participates in various bodily functions, including the breakdown of protein, the metabolism of carbohydrates, and the formation of fats.

A lack of this nutrient may produce seborrheic dermatitis, a skin rash often found in infants under six months of age. This condition may result in hair loss. Avidin, a type of protein found in uncooked egg whites, can prevent the absorption of biotin.

Note: A deficiency of biotin is rare because it can be manufactured in the intestines from other food.

Basic Nutritional Therapy

Supplements of biotin up to 100 *micro*grams per day may be taken by adults to ensure full benefits. My own position is that a good diet should provide plenty of this nutrient without supplementation. (See "Food Sources.")

Some exceptions noted in scientific literature include these:

- Infants under six months of age and some adults with seborrheic dermatitis.

- Kidney patients with nerve disorders resulting from their hemodialysis treatments. These patients have experienced relief of their neurological problems after biotin supplementation.

Special Food Sources, Strategies, and Facts

Here are some good food sources of biotin: soy flour, whole dry and nonfat dry milk, egg yolks, bananas, black currants, elderberries, grapes, cantaloupe, peaches, raisins, watermelon, beef liver (very high), lamb liver (very high), bacon (high), veal (high), almonds (high), peanuts (high), walnuts (high), perch, mushrooms, spinach, tomatoes.

Therapy Recommendations

Biotin is found in many foods, and so people who consume a variety of foods minimize the possibility of suffering a deficiency. Claims that biotin is needed in supplement form as a disease treatment or prevention are unfounded and misleading. Recommended daily intake of biotin has not been established.

Cross-References

See "Dermatitis."

VITAMIN C (ASCORBIC ACID)

Various scientific studies have shown that vitamin C may be helpful in preventing a number of diseases. (See "Basic Nutritional Therapy." Also, refer to Chapter 4 of this book.)

Although a considerable amount of vitamin C can be obtained through the diet, if you require doses in excess of 1,000 milligrams, you will almost certainly have to rely on supplements. (See "Basic Nutritional Therapy" and "Therapy Recommendations.")

Basic Nutritional Therapy

Relatively large doses of vitamin C (generally in excess of 1,000 milligrams daily) are associated with a number of health benefits:

- Enhancing the action of vitamin E in the body.
- Fighting the damage caused in the body by "free radicals," unstable oxygen molecules that can promote atherosclerosis, cancer, and a number of other serious diseases.
- Reducing the risk of heart disease.
- Reducing the risk of cancers of the stomach, esophagus, larynx, oral cavity, and pancreas.
- Reducing the risk of cataracts.
- Increasing immunity to infectious diseases.
- Possible lowering of total cholesterol and raising of "good" HDL cholesterol.
- Lowering high blood pressure.
- Promoting the healing of wounds, bodily growth, and tissue repair.

For more on nutritional therapy related to vitamin C, see Chapter 4.

Extra Scientific Information

- Vitamin C has been shown to help reduce the risk of cardiovascular disease, but the results with vitamin C have been less consistently positive than those with vitamin E, according to researchers reporting in the *Annals of Internal Medicine*, December 1, 1995, pp. 860-72.
- Men and women who consume two to three times the RDA for vitamin C (the RDA is 60 mg per day) have lower heart disease risk than those who consume less. Specifically, a study from the U.S. Department of Agriculture showed that the blood

levels of HDL cholesterol ("good" cholesterol) increased with greater intake of vitamin C. The increase was almost three times more in women over the age of fifty-eight than in younger women. Also, the rise was over four times more in men above fifty-eight than in younger men. But there was a limit to the response: The blood level of vitamin C did not increase with intakes above 215 mg of daily dietary intake of vitamin C by women, or 345 mg per day by men. (See *American Journal of Clinical Nutrition*, July 1994.)

- In animal studies conducted by I. Jialal and other researchers at the Center for Human Nutrition, University of Texas Southwestern Medical Center in Dallas, vitamin E showed considerable potency in countering oxidation of "bad" LDL cholesterol. Vitamin C, though less effective, was also found to reduce LDL oxidation.

Note: Oxidation of the LDL molecules has been linked to the buildup of plaque in the blood vessels during the process of atherosclerosis. (See *Canadian Journal of Cardiology*, October 1995 supplement, pp. 97G-103G.)

- A new skin cream, which contains 10 percent vitamin C and must be prescribed by a physician, is being used to reduce wrinkling and age spots. After using this cream for eight months, the participants showed significant improvement. Called "Cellox," it delivers 20-40 times the amount of vitamin C that can be absorbed from pills. (See *Health Confidential*, Vol. 10, no. 8, August 1996.)
- Most studies with vitamin C do not show any effect of the vitamin in preventing colds. But in several studies, 1,000-3,000 mg per day reduced the average duration of colds from six days to four and one-half

days. (See *Health Confidential*, Vol. 10, no. 8, August 1996.)

Special Food Sources, Strategies, and Facts

The highest food source of vitamin C is the acerola cherry from Barbados. One 8-ounce glass of fresh cherry juice contains more than 3,800 milligrams of vitamin C, and one cup of raw acerola fruit contains more than 1,600 milligrams of the nutrient.

Other sources high in vitamin C are: cranberry juice cocktail, guava, fresh orange juice, fresh grapefruit juice, papaya, red peppers, and strawberries. But to get just 500 to 550 milligrams each day from these sources, you would have to consume a total of one cup of strawberries, one papaya, one 8-ounce glass of orange juice, and one 8-ounce glass of cranberry juice cocktail. You can see the need for supplements to reach even the minimally required amounts that I recommend. (See "Therapy Recommendations.")

Therapy Recommendations

My recommendations for daily vitamin C consumption are as follows:

- Girls and young women five to twenty-one years of age: 200 mg daily
- Women twenty-two and older who are not heavy exercisers or overweight: 500 mg daily
- Women twenty-two and older who are heavy exercisers or weigh over 200 pounds: 1,000 mg daily
- Boys five to twelve years of age: 200 mg. daily
- Boys and young men thirteen to twenty-one years of age: 500 mg daily
- Men twenty-two to fifty who are not heavy exercisers or overweight: 1,000 mg daily

- Men over fifty years of age, who are not heavy exercisers or overweight: 1,500 mg daily
- Men over twenty-two years of age who are heavy exercisers or weigh over 200 pounds: 2,000 mg daily

For doses in the 500 milligram range, much of the daily vitamin C may be obtained through the diet. (See "Food Sources.") But in the higher ranges, above approximately 500 mg daily, supplements will be necessary.

Cross-References

See "Atherosclerosis," "Cancers," "Vitamin E," Chapter 4.

CAFFEINE

Caffeine, the mild stimulant found in coffee, tea, colas, chocolate, and a number of other beverages and foods, has a checkered history with regard to human health. In general, small amounts of caffeine each day seem to have no negative impact on health for most people and, in fact, may even be helpful. But the more caffeine you consume, the more your risks of health problems increase.

Basic Nutritional Therapy

In a study published in March 1996 in the American Medical Association's *Archives of Internal Medicine,* researchers at the Harvard Medical School reported that women who drink coffee are less likely to commit suicide than those who do not. Although the study has been criticized, it is consistent with another investigation conducted in 1993 by the Kaiser Permanente Medical Care Program, which found a lower risk of suicide among people who drink caffeine-containing beverages.

Also, a 1990 study on caffeine revealed that as little as 100 milligrams per day (less than one moderately strong cup of coffee) could increase feelings of well-being, energy, and motivation to work. One 5-ounce cup of brewed coffee (drip method) contains 100 to 150 milligrams of caffeine (average = 130 mg), according to the U.S. Food and Drug Administration. The range reflects variations in the strength of the coffee and the way it is prepared. For example, a 5-ounce cup of percolated coffee averages 94 mg of caffeine; a cup of instant coffee, 74 mg; and a cup of decaffeinated brewed or instant coffee, 3 mg.

Also on the positive side are numerous clinical and anecdotal reports that caffeine can improve mental acuity and, in some cases, athletic performance.

But there are also negatives associated with this stimulant in some people, especially when it is taken in large doses. These include:

- Raising of blood cholesterol with nonfiltered, boiled coffee.
- Aggravation of irritable bowel syndrome.
- Increasing symptoms associated with prostate infections.
- Magnified side effects, such as headaches or anxiety, when caffeine is combined with birth control pills.
- Shortness of breath.
- Headaches.
- Irregular heartbeat.
- Increased incidence of breast cysts in some women.
- Insomnia.
- Temporary elevation of blood pressure by five to fifteen mm of mercury. One French study showed a permanent increase in hypertension in patients who consumed five or more cups of coffee a day.
- Loss of the body's calcium through the urine, a result that could decrease bone density and lead to osteoporosis.
- Prevention of conception. A study at Johns Hopkins University, conducted in 1995 and reported in the

American Journal of Epidemiology, found that women who consume more than 300 milligrams of caffeine a day—about three cups of coffee (or eight caffeine-containing sodas)—reduce their chance of pregnancy by 26 percent.

Extra Scientific Information

- Nearly 50 percent of 288 men and women surveyed by University of Minnesota researchers said that they increase their consumption of coffee or caffeine-containing soft drinks when they are under stress, according to the July-August 1996 issue of *Addictive Behavior* (pp. 509-16). The most common reason they gave for taking in caffeine was the relief of stress.
- In animal studies conducted at the University of Karachi, Pakistan, caffeine withdrawal precipitated withdrawal symptoms, according to Life Sciences, September 29, 1995, pp. PL285-92.
- Caffeine alters the tone of coronary muscles while at rest, a condition that may make a heart disease patient more likely to experience shutoff of blood flow to the heart. (See the *Journal of Nuclear Medicine*, November 1995, pp. 2016-21.)
- Taken in doses commonly available in one cup of coffee, caffeine can significantly improve the therapeutic potential in humans of acetaminophen (the pain reliever in Tylenol®), concluded Pakistani researchers in *Biopharmacy and Drug Dispositions*, August 1995, pp. 481-7.
- Twenty-five managers who averaged daily caffeine consumption of 575 milligrams (about four to five cups of coffee per day) experienced increased systolic blood pressure during their caffeine intake, but their pressure went down shortly afterward. The managers also showed decreased effectiveness in

some aspects of their work when they were deprived of caffeine. (See *Psychopharmacology*, April 1995, pp. 377-84.)

- After reviewing the results of seventeen studies, researchers reported in the *Archives of Internal Medicine* that coffee, tea, and other beverages containing caffeine do not cause any persistent elevations in blood pressure. Even in people who do not consume caffeine on a regular basis, the blood pressure elevations that occur after caffeine consumption are short-lived, lasting only one day at most. But if noticeable heartbeat irregularities occur with caffeine intake, the substance must be avoided in all forms, including coffee, tea, colas, and chocolate.
- Among habitual coffee drinkers, improved cognitive performance occurred with higher levels of coffee consumption, but there was less of an improvement for tea drinkers, according to a study at the National Addiction Centre in London. Also, older people appeared to be more susceptible to the performance-improving effects of caffeine than were younger subjects. (See *Psychopharmacology*, 1993, pp. 45-52.)

Special Food Sources, Strategies, and Facts

Although precise amounts vary from cup to cup and food to food, you can assume approximately these average amounts of caffeine in common foods:

- 130 milligrams per 5-ounce cup of brewed, drip coffee
- 70 milligrams per 12-ounce glass of tea
- 50 milligrams per 5-ounce cup of brewed tea
- 40 milligrams per bottle or can of caffeine-containing soda
- 20 milligrams for every two squares of dark chocolate

Also, caffeine may be found in substantial quantities in over-the-counter medications and pills used to combat pain and sleepiness and to control weight. Examples per tablet: Excedrin®, 130 mg; Midol® and Anacin®, 65 mg; No Doz®, 200 mg; Dexatrim®, 200 mg.

Another important fact about caffeine already indicated in "Extra Scientific Information": The substance has the potential to be addictive. In the October 1994 *Journal of the American Medical Association*, research sponsored by the National Institute on Drug Abuse revealed that the main features of drug addiction could be found in certain people who consumed as little as one cup of coffee per day or as much as twenty-five cups. These features included (1) withdrawal symptoms when caffeine use was terminated; (2) development of tolerance over time to the effects of caffeine; (3) use of caffeine in spite of aggravation of medical or mental problems; and (4) repeated, unsuccessful efforts to quit using it.

Therapy Recommendations

If caffeine is a part of your daily routine, there is usually no need to eliminate it completely, unless your physician prohibits it for specific health reasons.

If you do take in caffeine, at least follow this minimal guideline, which many medical experts observe: Limit your daily consumption to a milligram amount that is no more than double your body weight in pounds. So if you weigh 120 pounds, you should take in no more than 240 milligrams of caffeine per day. That translates to about two cups of moderately strong coffee each day.

I go even further in my personal recommendations to my patients. I urge that *everyone,* regardless of weight, limit intake of caffeine to no more than two cups of coffee or tea per day.

Cross-References

See "Cholesterol," "Heart Disease."

CALCIUM

Adequate levels of calcium in the diet are essential for strong bones and teeth, and also for a variety of other important body functions, including the work of enzymes in the digestive tract. This mineral plays an especially important role in protecting aging men and women from osteoporosis, the bone-weakening disease that affects an estimated 24 million Americans.

Basic Nutritional Therapy

The 1994 recommendation from the National Institutes of Health for calcium is 1,000 milligrams per day for adults, with the amount being increased to 1,500 milligrams per day for women who are pregnant or nursing a child. Women over fifty on estrogen should get 1,000 mg, while those not on estrogen should receive 1,500 mg. Men and women over sixty-five should take in 1,500 mg per day. I believe these amounts are adequate to ensure protection against most osteoporosis. As a result, I urge that everyone take a minimum of 1,000 milligrams of calcium per day, with pregnant and lactating women and very active people ingesting closer to 1,500 milligrams. (See "Therapy Recommendations.")

If possible, you should get all of your calcium from foods (see "Food Sources"), but this may be difficult, especially if you have trouble digesting dairy products. A significant percent of the world's population is unable to eat dairy foods because of stomach and intestinal problems, such as cramps or gas. These are due to a condition known as "lactose intolerance," or a lack of the enzyme lactase, which is necessary to digest the lactose sugars in milk.

For people with lactose intolerance or some other aversion to dairy products, calcium supplements are a must. Most often, calcium supplements are taken in one of the following forms: calcium carbonate, calcium phosphate, calcium gluconate, or calcium citrate. (See "Therapy Recommendations.")

Note: Various studies have shown that increasing calcium in the diet or through supplements works particularly well when the mineral is combined with regular exercise or as part of estrogen replacement therapy. Estrogen replacement therapy may be recommended for a number of reasons, including protection against osteoporosis and heart disease for women who have gone through menopause. By taking estrogen after menopause, women may be able to lower their "bad" cholesterol (LDL) and raise their "good" cholesterol (HDL). (For more on this subject, see "Hormones" entry.)

To be absorbed in the body and used in bone growth, calcium needs the help of vitamin D, which becomes available to the human system through exposure to sunlight or supplements. Most people get plenty of vitamin D just by being outdoors a half hour every day. But for elderly or sick shut-ins, vitamin D supplementation may be required.

Caution: Use vitamin D supplements *only* under the supervision of a physician. While a maximum of 400 IUs (international units) is required each day, overdoses can actually cause the destruction of bones or other problems.

In addition to helping in the fight against osteoporosis and cardiovascular disease, calcium has a number of other important uses. For example, scientists at the Arizona Cancer Center reported in January 1996 in the *Journal of the National Cancer Institute,* that a diet high in calcium could lower the risk of cancer of the colon by 35 percent. The participants in the study, who consumed 1,500 milligrams of calcium supplements per day, probably lowered their risk because of the tendency of calcium to soak up acids that stimulate the growth of malignant tumors.

There are also studies indicating that calcium may help lower blood pressure in some people, particularly pregnant women. But other findings suggest the opposite, that calcium can actually raise blood pressure. As a result, if you have hypertension, it's wise to consult your physician before you take extra calcium. (See more on this topic under "Extra Scientific Information.")

Extra Scientific Information

- In animal studies at the Oregon Health Sciences University in 1995, researchers found that supplemental dietary calcium lowered blood pressure, while restricted calcium diets tended to elevate blood pressure. (See *Seminars in Nephrology*, November 1995, pp. 593-602.)
- In humans, low dietary intake of calcium has been found to be a risk factor for hypertension in a number of epidemiological studies, according to French scientists reporting in the November 1995 issue of *Seminars in Nephrology* (pp. 550-63). Increased dietary calcium intake seems to have a beneficial influence on blood pressure in humans.
- In contrast, researchers at the Oregon Health Sciences University report that the role of calcium in preventing or treating hypertension remains unclear. For one thing, the results are inconclusive because of variations of methodologies in the different studies. Also, some people at risk for hypertension may be helped by the intake of calcium, while others may not. The medical community needs to focus on ways to identify patients who may be helped most by additional calcium.
- An animal study conducted at the University of

Illinois demonstrated that spinach suppresses calcium absorption in the bones of young animals. As a result, there was a reduction in both the quality and quantity of the bone. Spinach, though high in calcium, is regarded as "a low in bioavailability calcium source." In other words, it's hard for our enzymes and digestive juices to "unlock" calcium in spinach for use in the body. (See *Journal of the American College of Nutrition*, June 1995, pp. 278-85.)

- A 1995 Japanese study showed that a calcium dietary supplement could be used to help prevent pregnancy-induced hypertension. Only 2.2 percent of the pregnant women who took 1 gram of calcium per day developed hypertension. This finding contrasted with 8.8 percent hypertensives in the non-calcium group. (See *Journal of Obstetrics and Gynecology*, June 1995, pp. 281-88.)

- There is an important discrepancy between perceived and actual calcium intake, according to researchers at the University of Illinois. (See the *Journal of American College of Nutrition*, August 1995, pp. 336-40.) Researchers found that the mean calcium intake of the more than 300 women surveyed was 591 milligrams per day. Also, over 40 percent of the women reported intakes below 60 percent of the National Institutes of Health's recommendation for calcium (1,000 mg per day). Yet among those with a deficient intake of calcium, 27 percent believed they were meeting the calcium RDA.

Special Food Sources, Strategies, and Facts

The best dairy sources of dietary calcium, with milligram amounts indicated, are:

- Skim and low-fat milk (300-325 mg in an 8-ounce glass)

- Yogurt, plain and low-fat (415 mg per cup)
- Ricotta cheese (340 mg per 1/2 cup)
- Swiss cheese (270 mg per ounce)
- Monterey, provolone, cheddar, Gouda cheese (200-214 mg per ounce)
- American and mozzarella cheese (150-180 mg per ounce)

Some good nondairy sources include sardines with bones (324 mg per 3-ounce can in oil); canned salmon with bones (180 mg per 3-ounce can); tofu (108 mg per 3 ounces); frozen, cooked collards (179 mg per 1/2 cup); frozen, boiled kale (90 mg per 1/2 cup); frozen, chopped broccoli (94 mg per 1/2 cup).

Therapy Recommendations

Every adult and teenager should take in 1,000 to 1,500 milligrams of calcium per day. Pregnant, lactating, and postmenopausal women, as well as very active individuals and athletes who perspire a great deal, should lean toward the upper end of this range.

Children also need plenty of calcium. The RDA requirements for young people, with which I generally agree, are:

- Infants up to six months of age: 400 mg per day
- Infants six to twelve months: 600 mg per day
- Children one to five years of age: 800 mg per day
- Children six to ten years of age: 800-1,200 mg per day
- Children and young adults: eleven to twenty-four years: 1,200 mg per day (I would suggest an upper ceiling of 1,500)

If you can get your entire dose of calcium through your daily diet, you won't need to rely on supplements. But if you can't reach the above calcium requirements from your food, then you should get the remaining portion through supplementation. Many good products are now on the market, but be sure to look beyond the brand names to see that the bottle contains one of these calcium compounds:

- Calcium carbonate (the most common supplement, found in such products as Os-Cal®)
- Calcium phosphate (generally thought to be less bioavailable than the carbonate form)
- Calcium gluconate (absorbed easily by most people, but containing little calcium in comparison with other tablets; consequently, you have to take more)
- Calcium citrate (has high bioavailability)

Be sure to check the bottle to ascertain the number of milligrams of calcium in each tablet. The amount of calcium will vary greatly from product to product.

To promote better absorption into your system, it's best to take calcium supplements in small doses one hour before meals or two hours after a meal. Also, various studies have shown that absorption is enhanced among people who are involved in regular weight-bearing, endurance exercise, such as jogging, walking, or cycling.

Cross-References

See "Cholesterol," "Heart Disease," "High Blood Pressure," "Hormones," "Osteoporosis."

CANCERS

Cancer, which is gaining rapidly on heart disease as the leading cause of death among Americans, often tends to run in families. Inherited or environmental predispositions can make one person more susceptible to this killer than another person.

But your genes and background do not necessarily determine your destiny with cancer. Taking certain preventive steps, especially consuming an anticancer diet, can lower anyone's risk significantly. This section provides an overview of how you can protect yourself against cancer. Other parts of this book, including the sections mentioned in the "Cross-References" and other subsections under this entry, give more details about specific cancer-fighting foods and strategies.

Basic Nutritional Therapy

To protect yourself against cancer, follow these nutritional steps:

1. Cut down on fats, especially saturated fats. (See "Fat.") Specifically, limit your intake of saturated fats to less than 8 percent of your daily intake of calories.

2. Increase your intake of fruits, vegetables, and whole grains. Various studies have shown that vegetarians tend to have a lower incidence of cancer.

Dozens of studies have found that a diet weighted heavily in favor of vegetables is correlated with a low risk of cancer. Also, people consuming a higher intake of carotenoids have a lower risk of lung cancer. Apparently, it's the carotenoids or other closely associated substances in plants that help distinguish those who are going to get lung cancer from those who will not. (See *American Journal of Clinical Nutrition*, 1994, 1162S-5S.)

3. Eat plenty of fiber, especially insoluble fiber. (See "Fiber, Insoluble.") You can help to prevent cancer by eating both soluble fiber (fiber that dissolves in water, such as the fibers in oatmeal and citrus fruits) and insoluble fiber (the type that will *not* dissolve in water, such as cellulose

fibers in wheat bran). For the strongest protection against cancer, your emphasis should be on the insoluble type.

A diet high in fiber (at least 20 to 35 grams per day) can significantly lower your risk of cancers of the breast, stomach, colon, female sexual organs, and the oral cavity.

4. Take in extra amounts of the antioxidants vitamin C, vitamin E, and beta-carotene. (See Chapter 4 of this book and page 127 of my *Antioxidant Revolution* for specific recommendations and doses.)

Vitamin C lowers the risk of cancers of the stomach, esophagus, larynx, oral cavity, and pancreas. Vitamin E has been linked to reduced risk of a number of cancers, including those of the prostate, colon, and rectum. Studies have associated beta-carotene with protection against cancers of the esophagus, bladder, rectum, skin (melanoma), and lung.

Note: Folic acid, or folate, discussed briefly as an entry in Part II and more extensively in Chapters 2 and 3, has been linked in some studies to a decreased incidence of rectal cancer, colon cancer, and colon adenomas.

5. Minimize your intake of cured, pickled, and smoked foods. Pickled vegetables, potatoes, salted fish, and abrasive food grains have been related to an increase in stomach cancers.

6. Minimize the use of foods heavy in hormones and contaminants that are associated with cancer. In particular, the use of hormones in food processing may be a factor in common hormone-related cancers such as those of the breast, uterus, and prostate. Other potentially carcinogenic materials include pesticide residues, agricultural chemicals, and products of fuel combustion and cooking.

7. If you consume alcoholic beverages, your intake should be moderate. (See "Alcohol" entry.)

Special Food Sources, Strategies, and Facts

You should try to get most of your nutritional protection from cancer through your diet. This means eating plenty of fruits, vegetables, and whole grain products—the primary sources of cancer-fighting fiber and antioxidants (especially vitamin C and beta-carotene). Cruciferous vegetables, particularly cauliflower, brussels sprouts, cabbage, broccoli, and onions are powerful anticancer agents. Tomatoes and tomato products seem to provide some protection from prostate cancer.

Because of the difficulty of getting all the antioxidants you need through your food, it will probably be necessary to supplement your diet with vitamin C and beta-carotene (see Chapter 4). Vitamin E supplements are also a must because of the impossibility of taking in enough of this nutrient through your food. (See "Cross-References.")

Therapy Recommendations

The nutritional steps listed under "Basic Nutritional Therapy" sum up my basic recommendations. Details on antioxidant doses and other specific concerns are in Chapter 4 of this book and also in the entries listed under "Cross-References."

Cross-References

See "Vitamin A," "Cruciferous Vegetables," "Vitamin E," "Fat," "Fiber, Insoluble," "Fiber, Soluble," "Meat."

CARBOHYDRATES

Carbohydrates, one of the three main components of your diet along with protein and fats, represent the most readily available and powerful form of energy for the body. The more energy you require every day, the more carbohydrates you should plug into your diet.

In general, you should get at least 50 to 70 percent of the calories that you consume every day from *complex* carbohydrates; about 10 to 20 percent from protein-rich foods; and 20 to 30 percent from fats (with no more than one-third of your fat calories coming from saturated fats). (See the "Fat" entry.)

By "complex carbohydrates" I mean those highly nutritional foods like fruits, vegetables, and starches (such as potatoes), which consist mainly of complex carbon-hydrogen-oxygen molecules. I'm *not* referring to *simple* carbohydrates such as table sugar, candy, or other sweets. The body's energy systems make much better and longer-lasting use of complex carbohydrates than they do of simple sugars.

Basic Nutritional Therapy

A high percentage of complex carbohydrates, at least 50 to 70 percent of total daily calories, is necessary for the nutritional fuel you need to perform your daily activities efficiently. These foods provide most of the natural vitamins, minerals, and other nutrients you require.

Complex carbohydrates are also our main source of fiber, and this is a major factor in reducing the risk of cancer, heart disease, diverticulitis, and many other diseases. (See "Fiber, Soluble," and "Fiber, Insoluble.")

Most complex carbohydrates contain a high proportion of water. To keep your body's systems functioning properly, including the bowels and urinary tract, you should take in the equivalent of at least eight 8-ounce glasses of fluid every day. Since you probably won't reach this goal just by drinking tap water, you need to rely on fruits and other complex carbohydrates to meet your quota.

Although the average person can get along by taking in 50 to 70 percent of daily calories from complex carbohydrates, you may need more if you are a *very* active person or have a particularly high metabolism. If you engage in some relatively strenuous form of athletics, you may want to increase the percentage of carbohydrates by 10 percent or more. There are two ways to do this.

You can simply increase the percentage of carbohydrates you consume every day. You may find that you operate better when you take in 65 or even 70 percent of your calories from complex carbohydrates on a regular basis.

If you are an adult who engages in strenuous athletic competitions, or must engage in other periodic high-energy-demand activities, you may want to try a form of "carbohydrate loading" before the demanding event.

Carbohydrate loading is a practice pioneered by endurance runners and now used by many athletes to increase fuel stores in the body. The idea is to pack the muscles with glycogen, the sugar used by the body to produce maximum energy and performance during a sports event.

There have been many theories on how to do this. One ill-considered concept involved totally depleting the muscles of glycogen a few days before an event and then packing in huge amounts of pasta and other complex carbohydrates to restore the lost glycogen. The idea was that by cleaning out your system you could actually increase the capacity of the muscles to store glycogen. But most experts now feel that this approach may actually backfire by weakening the body too much.

A healthier and safer approach is just to increase the intake of carbohydrates to about 70 to 75 percent of total calories, beginning three to four days before the event. This way, your body can produce plenty of extra glycogen without upsetting your basic nutritional balance.

Note: I don't believe that children or teenage athletes should engage in this loading practice. It's quite all right for them to eat high amounts of carbohydrates on a regular basis, in the 60 to 65 percent range of total calories. But growing bones, muscles, nerves, and brain tissue also require plenty of protein-rich foods and some unsaturated fats. Frequent carbohydrate loading during a particular sports season may cause a young person to skimp on the necessary protein and fat, often with disastrous results.

Extra Scientific Information

- Carbohydrate ingestion while exercising is necessary to sustain prolonged exercise of low to moderate intensity, according to a report on trained cyclists from the University of Cape Town Medical School in Observatory, South Africa (*Pflugers Archives*, October 1995, pp. 971-7). All the cyclists who took in carbohydrates finished a three-hour continuous trial session. But one-third of another group of cyclists, who were given only flavored water, failed to finish the test.
- A reduced fat diet, enriched by carbohydrates and oleic acids (a monounsaturated fat found in such foods as olive oil), can result in significant improvements in the fatty (lipid) content in the blood. (See *Arctic Medical Research*, October 1995, pp. 160-9.)
- Researchers at McMaster University Medical Center in Hamilton, Ontario, Canada, compared the ability of male and female endurance athletes to increase their muscle glycogen (sugar) concentrations in response to carbohydrate loading. The loading regimen involved increasing their dietary carbohydrate intake from 55 to 60 percent of their daily calories to 75 percent of their calories, for a period of four days.

(See *Journal of Applied Physiology*, April 1995, pp. 1360-8.)

The results: The men increased their muscle glycogen concentrations by 41 percent and had a corresponding increase in their performance times. In contrast, the women did not increase their glycogen concentrations or their performance times. The researchers concluded that, at least in this particular test, women were unable to increase their muscle glycogen as much as men in response to carbohydrate loading.

- Increasing carbohydrate intake of endurance-trained cyclists by 72 percent for three days prior to an exercise trial produced a number of effects: (1) the pre-exercise muscle glycogen in the cyclists increased; (2) their power output improved; and (3) they extended the distance they were able to cover, in contrast to their distances when on a lower carbohydrate diet. (See *International Journal of Sports Nutrition*, March 1995, pp. 25-36.)

Special Food Sources, Strategies, and Facts

Nutritious foods high in complex carbohydrates include: fresh vegetables (focus on such foods as broccoli, carrots, cabbage, brussels sprouts, cauliflower, sweet potatoes); fresh fruits (focus on citrus fruits, cantaloupe, fresh juices, apples); potatoes; rice; beans; peas; lentils; corn; pasta; whole grain breads and cereals; and cereal brans.

Note: This list is *not* meant to be exhaustive. There are plenty of other fruits, vegetables, and whole grain foods that can provide you with the complex carbohydrate levels you need each day. Also, the foods suggested above represent some of *my* personal favorites that I know will give me not only high-powered carbohydrate energy, but also the vitamins and minerals I need.

To come up with a ballpark percentage for the number of complex carbohydrate calories you consume each day, try this approach:

First find the caloric value of a particular food portion. You can get this information in any listing of caloric values in various nutrition reference books available in your library or bookstore. Examples are the *Handbook of the Nutritional Contents of Foods,* which is prepared for the U.S. Department of Agriculture, or *Bowes & Church's Food Values of Portions Commonly Used.*

After you have found the caloric values of the high-carbohydrate foods in your diet, make these general assumptions about carbohydrate vs. protein percentages:

- Whole fruit usually contains about 95 percent carbohydrate and 5 percent protein.
- Fruit juice usually contains about 97 percent carbohydrate and 3 percent protein.
- Vegetables usually contain about 60 percent carbohydrate and 40 percent protein.
- Vegetable juice usually contains about 80 percent carbohydrate and 20 percent protein.
- Whole grain cereals usually contain about 80 percent carbohydrate and 20 percent protein. However, there is a wide variation, depending on the contents and fortified nature of the cereal. Whenever possible, check the carbohydrate and protein values on the box labels.

Now, do these simple calculations:

Your calorie listing might show that one cup of cooked oatmeal contains about 145 calories. Multiply that by 80 percent (0.80), which is the approximate carbohydrate value of many cereals. That will give you 116 calories from carbohydrate. (The exact value is closer to 110 calories of carbohydrate, but your figure is close enough.)

It's helpful to figure out the carbohydrate values in all your menus for several days in a row so that you can ascertain what percentage of your diet consists of carbohydrates. (Obviously, it's also important to perform the same exercise for protein and fat. For help, see the discussions under "Amino Acids" and "Fat.")

I also suggest that you figure out the carbohydrate values for your favorite foods and then write them down on a master list for later reference. Soon, you'll know approximately what carbohydrate caloric values and percentages most of your foods contain. That will help you estimate the percentage of carbohydrates you are taking in each day.

An alternative method for the scientists among us: If you want to figure out more precisely the number of calories generated by carbohydrates in your diet, you should first find the number of grams of carbohydrate in the particular food. To do this, use the listings found in the reference books and other sources mentioned above.

Next, you should know that 1 gram of carbohydrate produces about 4 calories. With this information at hand, you are ready to do some *real* calculations.

Suppose you are wondering about the carbohydrate calories in the oranges you eat. Using your food-table listings, you will find that one average-size orange contains about 15 grams of carbohydrate. Also, the total number of calories in an orange is 62. It takes only some simple math to see that the number of calories attributable to the carbohydrate content is 60 (15 grams times 4 calories per gram equals 60 calories). The percentage of carbohydrate calories in an orange, then, is 96 percent.

You can use a similar approach to find the overall percentage of your daily calories coming from carbohydrates. Just identify all the foods you consume on a given day; add up the total calories you take in; add the carbohydrate calories; and then find the percentage represented by the carbohydrates.

You may find that your total daily calorie intake is 2,800 calories, of which 1,550 calories come from carbohydrates. This means that you are getting 55 percent of your calories from carbohydrates (divide 1,550 by 2,800 and then multiply the quotient by 100 to get the percentage).

However you do the calculations, you should try to get a grasp on the percentage of carbohydrate calories you are consuming each day. That's one of the best ways I know to keep your energy levels high, your intake of important nutrients healthy, and your overall food program in balance.

Therapy Recommendations

If you have average energy needs, set a target of getting 60 percent of your calories every day from foods high in complex carbohydrates.

If you are engaging actively in sports or you lead a high-energy life, increase your complex carbohydrate calories to 65 to 70 percent of your daily intake.

In trying to establish the optimum amount for your body, use this self-diagnosis: If you find that your level of activity leaves you feeling somewhat fatigued or irritable, increase your intake of complex carbohydrates gradually until your energy returns.

If you reach the 75 percent level and still feel fatigued or out of sorts, see your physician for an evaluation. Your physical problems are probably the result of some nonnutritional factor, such as too little sleep, overtraining, excessive stress, or perhaps an underlying health condition or disease.

Cross-References

See "Amino Acids," "Fat," "Fiber, Insoluble," "Fiber, Soluble," "Ketogenic Diet," "Protein."

CARPAL TUNNEL SYNDROME

Carpal tunnel syndrome is a condition that may afflict typists, keypunch operators, musicians, and others who engage in extensive, repetitive hand movements. Symptoms include pain, numbness, tingling, burning, or other discomfort in the nerves in the middle of the hand or the thumb region.

Basic Nutritional Therapy

The primary ways to treat this problem include rest, splinting, physiotherapy, and surgery. But nutritional therapy may also be of help. Supplements of pyridoxine (vitamin B_6) have helped some patients find relief.

Caution: Don't try to doctor yourself for this condition. Check with your physician about the possibility of vitamin therapy.

Extra Scientific Information

- A study at the Department of Neurology, Kaiser Permanente Medical Center in Hayward, California, revealed that the pain of patients with mild to moderate carpal tunnel syndrome was reduced following vitamin B_6 (pyridoxine) treatment. (See *Journal of American College of Nutrition*, February 1993, pp. 73-6.) A daily dosage of 200 mg of pyridoxine was used for three months without significant side effects. Pain scores during patient interviews improved dramatically and accurately predicted return of physical function. Investigators noted that the cause of improvement might have been that the vitamin B_6 raised the pain thresholds of the patients.

A University of Michigan study concluded that physicians who prescribe vitamin B_6 for those who suffer from carpal tunnel syndrome could be doing their patients more harm than good. Standard treatment includes wearing splints, taking anti-inflammatory drugs, modifying activities, and using physical therapy.

After studying 125 employees of two auto parts plants, the investigators could find no relationship between blood levels of vitamin B_6 and the carpal tunnel syndrome symptoms. But the researchers made no attempt in the study to treat those employees who had classic symptoms. (See *Journal of Occupational and Environmental Medicine*, May 1996.)

- In a study conducted at the Department of Family Medicine, University of Alberta, Edmonton, Canada, findings did not support the use of vitamin B_6 for treatment of carpal tunnel syndrome. (See *Canadian Family Physician*, October 1993, pp. 2122-7.) The researchers examined the effect of the vitamin on thirty-two patients but found no clinical or electrical signs, nor any significant symptoms of the condition.
- Vitamin B_6 supplements may help patients with carpal tunnel syndrome, according to a letter printed in the June 10, 1995, issue of the *British Medical Journal* (p. 1534).

Special Food Sources, Strategies, and Facts

For foods high in pyridoxine (vitamin B_6) see "Vitamin B_6."

Therapy Recommendations

Treatment of carpal tunnel syndrome with pyridoxine supplements has involved varying amounts of the vitamin. Although you should not try to treat yourself, do feel free to suggest the nutritional therapy approach to your physician.

Cross-References

See "Vitamin B_6."

CATARACTS

There is evidence that cataracts, the clouding of the lens of the eye from age-related thickening, frequently occurs in the older person, and may result in blindness. Nutritional therapy may be of value in preventing or delaying this problem.

This condition is thought to be caused by the ravages of free radicals in the body, including those triggered by exposure to sunlight. Viral infections, exposure to toxic substances, and genetic disorders also cause cataracts. By some estimates, nearly half of the elderly population over age seventy-five suffers from cataracts. If the problem is not surgically corrected, visual impairment can occur.

The condition has been linked to possible excess sugar intake and to deficiencies of riboflavin, vitamin C, vitamin E, selenium, or zinc.

Nutrition's strongest connection with cataracts lies in the role of antioxidants, such as carotenoids, vitamin C, and vitamin E, all of which may help prevent cataracts. One study compared supplement use by 175 people who had cataracts, with 175 matched controls. The researchers found that those who had no cataracts took significantly more supplements of vitamins C and E than those who did have cataracts.

Three hundred milligrams or more of vitamin C daily,

taken over a long period of time, may lower the risk of cataracts by up to 70 percent. Also, daily supplements of 400 IU of vitamin E may cut cataract risk in half, and combining E and C may be even more beneficial. The B vitamin riboflavin may also be beneficial by helping the body maximize its antioxidant defenses. (See "Basic Nutritional Therapy" below, as well as the more extensive treatment of antioxidants in Chapter 4.)

Basic Nutritional Therapy

There is no guarantee that changing your diet will eliminate your risk of getting cataracts. But a growing body of studies suggests that the basic "antioxidant cocktail," which I recommended in my *Antioxidant Revolution* and in an updated version in Chapter 3 of this book, could provide significant protection.

Studies suggest that men should take in at least 500 milligrams of vitamin C daily, and women should have a minimum of 200 milligrams per day. Other data suggest that protection from cataracts can come from vitamin E, beta-carotene, and bioflavonoids, which are present in the white covering of peeled oranges as well as in other fruits, buckwheat, and other foods. (See "Bioflavonoids.")

Also, animal studies have established that a diet deficient in riboflavin (vitamin B_2) can cause cataracts. (See "Vitamin B_2.")

As far as humans are concerned, the Linxian China study found a significant protective effect for nuclear cataracts in people who received riboflavin and niacin, compared with those not receiving these vitamins. The oldest subgroup in the study, those ages sixty-four to seventy-four years, benefited the most from the treatment with a 44 percent reduction in prevalence of cataracts. (See *Archives of Ophthalmology*, Vol. 111, September 1993.)

Finally, daily intake of alcohol is associated with a

modest increase in the risk of cataracts. And a few cases have linked congenital cataracts to a vitamin D deficiency.

Special Food Sources, Strategies, and Facts

For a listing of foods that can help to counter cataracts, see the food listings in the entries listed under "Cross-References."

Therapy Recommendations

To lower your risk of cataracts, get as many of the basic antioxidant vitamins as you can through your food, including vitamin C, vitamin E, and beta-carotene. To this end, consider taking my updated "antioxidant cocktail" described in Chapter 4 and also in my *Antioxidant Revolution*, page 127. For adults, I recommend a minimum of 500 to 1,000 milligrams of vitamin C each day, a minimum of 400 to 800 IUs of vitamin E, and a minimum of 25,000 IUs of beta-carotene (for nonsmokers).

Cross-References

See "Vitamin A," "Vitamin B$_2$," "Bioflavonoids," "Vitamin C," "Vitamin E."

CHILI PEPPERS

The medicinal properties of chili peppers, also referred to as "cayenne pepper" and "red pepper," were known to many ancient peoples, including the Aztecs. This hot plant food is known technically as "capsicum" and contains an alkaloidal ingredient, "capsaicin." It can reduce pain and other discomforts in a number of ways. For example, chili peppers and their extracts have been used to relieve peptic ulcers, arthritis, mouth sores, itching feet, skin irritations, and various diabetic symptoms.

Basic Nutritional Therapy

If you experience any of the pains and discomforts mentioned above, add some chili peppers to your diet.

But heed this warning: Exposing your skin to the powerful chemicals in peppers can produce painful inflammation and sores and, in some instances, may even result in death. (See "Extra Scientific Information.")

Extra Scientific Information

- Capsaicin, the pungent ingredient of chili, can protect against aspirin-induced damage to the stomach lining, according to a study conducted at the National University Hospital in Singapore. (See *Digest of Discoveries in Science*, March 1995, pp. 580-3.)

- Researchers at the National University of Singapore found that chili use has a protective effect against peptic ulcer disease. (See *Digest of Discoveries in Science*, March 1995, pp. 576-9.)

- A sixty-six-year-old man experienced painful sores on both hands as a result of having prepared and pickled fifteen quarts of homegrown jalapeño peppers. (See *Cutis*, February 1993, pp. 112-4.)

- An over-the-counter product containing capsaicin, which was used to treat neuralgia, diabetic pains, and arthritis discomforts, caused contact dermatitis (inflammation and itching of the skin) in a patient studied at the University of California-San Diego Medical Center. (See *Annals of Emerging Medicine*, May 1995, pp. 713-5.)

- The use of a mace-type pepper spray to control criminal suspects has been associated with possible deaths of prison inmates, according to research at the Department of Pathology, Bowman Gray School of Medicine, in Winston-Salem, North Carolina. (See

American Journal of Forensic Medical Pathology, September 1995, pp. 185-92.)
- Some claims have been made that capsaicin is effective in lowering blood cholesterol and preventing the clotting of blood. Yet there is a lack of supporting evidence.

Still, capsaicin ointment (Zostrix® and Axsain®), applied topically, has been used effectively to treat the chronic pain associated with shingles (Herpes zoster), trigeminal neuralgia, and trauma from surgical procedures. This ointment may also be of value in treating cluster headaches and pain associated with rheumatoid arthritis, diabetes, neuralgia that follows a bout with herpes, and pain that follows a mastectomy.

Special Food Sources, Strategies, and Facts

Any hot pepper contains the healthful ingredient capsaicin, which may produce the above results. These peppers also contain significant amounts of vitamin A, vitamin C, and potassium.

Therapy Recommendations

Get in the habit of using chili peppers occasionally in dips and for seasoning of your foods.

When you are experiencing pain or discomfort from arthritis or any of the conditions mentioned above, try consuming chili peppers daily. But be careful not to handle these peppers extensively during food preparation, and don't get the juice in your eyes!

Cross-References

See "Vitamin A," "Vitamin C."

CHOCOLATE

We most often think of chocolate as a source of guilty pleasures. The "chocoholics" among us are constantly fighting off the urge to eat too much of this sweet. But taken in reasonable doses, chocolate may actually be an aid in lowering cholesterol, elevating a "down" mood, and even fighting alcoholism. Some of these effects may be from caffeine, but actually, there is very little in chocolate. One ounce has only 5 mg of caffeine, an amount comparable to one cup of decaffeinated coffee.

Basic Nutritional Therapy

There is evidence in various scientific studies that chocolate has the power to:

* Raise "good" HDL cholesterol but *not* elevate "bad" LDL cholesterol. Even though chocolate is high in saturated fat, usually a cause of increasing bad cholesterol, the sweet also contains stearic acid, which is thought to be an agent that keeps cholesterol under control.
* Diminish an alcoholic's desire to drink.
* Relieve depression and pain by increasing serotonin, and stimulate physical and mental powers probably through the increase in endorphins, neurotransmitters in the brain that have been called the body's own morphine. The reason for this power in chocolate may be the presence of the stimulants caffeine and theobromine. Chocolate contains amine compounds called tyramine and phenylethylamine (PEA), which stimulate the metabolism.

But in some people, chocolate may have a number of negative effects. For example, it can aggravate high blood pressure, obesity (through "chocolate addiction"), symptoms of diabetes mellitus, kidney stones, low blood sugar after a meal (postprandial hypoglycemia), or a tendency to have irregular heartbeats. In some people, chocolate can also trigger headaches, especially migraines, as it dilates blood vessels in the brain. In others, it may aggravate heartburn by causing reflux of acids from the stomach into the esophagus. If you have any of these conditions, be sure that you consult your physician before you make chocolate a part of your diet.

Extra Scientific Information

- In a 1994 study at Pennsylvania State University, eating one milk chocolate bar per day for twenty-seven days raised the participants' high-density lipoproteins (HDL or "good" cholesterol) but did not affect the low-density lipoproteins (LDL or "bad" cholesterol). Researchers surmised that this response was due to the beneficial effect of stearic acid on the cholesterol. (See *American Journal of Clinical Nutrition*, December 1994, 6 Supplement, pp. 1037S-42S.)

- Animal studies conducted at the School of Medicine, East Carolina University, Greenville, North Carolina, revealed that a chocolate drink, tomato juice, and other fluids suppressed the desire to drink alcohol. (See *Physiologic Behavior*, June 1995, pp. 1155-61.)

- You may have strongly suspected this, but finally, here is solid scientific proof: Although chocolate provides pleasure, people who regard eating the sweet as an excessive or forbidden delight experience only short-lived pleasure, quickly followed by feelings of guilt. (See *British Journal of Clinical Psychology*, February 1995, pp. 129-38.)

- Researchers at Princess Margaret Hospital for Children in Perth, Australia, devised an edible chocolate spacer device for two young asthmatics to use as a bronchodilator. The investigators found that the chocolate spacer produced a significantly improved respiratory response in the two children. But in a related test, a regular, nonchocolate spacer produced no significant response. (See *Medical Journal of Australia*, December 4, 1995, pp. 587-8.)

Special Food Sources, Strategies, and Facts

Cacao, the South American tree seed that is the primary ingredient in chocolate, has been consumed since about A.D. 460. In the sixteenth century, explorer and conquistador Hernando Cortés took a bitter drink of *chocolat* from the court of the Aztec king Montezuma back to Spain. Soon, the popularity of the brew spread over Europe, but the candy version didn't develop until the nineteenth century, when the cocoa press was invented.

Per capita consumption of chocolate candy in the United States is relatively moderate (about 4.6 kilograms per year) as compared with that of many northern European countries (about 7 to 10 kilograms per year). Still, 11 percent of the U.S. population reported consuming chocolate candy in at least one of the three days when the overall national food intake was recorded by the U.S. Department of Agriculture in 1987-88 (the Nationwide Food Consumption Survey). (See *American Journal of Clinical Nutrition*, December 1994, 6 Supplement, pp. 1060S-4S.)

A few more facts:

- The western part of the United States has the highest proportion of American chocolate consumers.
- More whites than other racial groups use the sweet.
- Winter is the favorite season to eat it.

Chocolate has also been identified as the food most desired by women who binge. Men, in contrast, have the highest craving for snack foods high in fat and salt.

According to a report in the July 1995 issue of *American Journal of Clinical Nutrition*, the brain naturally produces opiate-like chemicals (endorphins) that cause pleasurable sensations linked to many addictions. But when the production of those "pleasure chemicals" is blocked, the urge to overeat chocolate declines.

In the study conducted by University of Michigan nutritionists, a group of women were given injections of naloxone (a drug used to treat heroin overdoses). Then they were offered chocolate chip cookies, chocolate ice cream, and similar sweets. The drug made the bingers in the group eat significantly less chocolate than they normally did.

Therapy Recommendations

If you have a cholesterol problem and you absolutely must have some sweets every day, chocolate is probably your best choice. But limit yourself each day to a couple of small, pure chocolate squares (not filled candies or chocolate mixed with other dessert material). Any more sweets, even including extra doses of pure chocolate, may drive up your weight and could have a negative effect on your total cholesterol.

Caution: If you have a problem with hypertension, obesity, diabetes mellitus, kidney stones, postmeal hypoglycemia, or irregular heartbeats, check with your physician before you include chocolate in your diet.

Cross-References

See "Cholesterol Regulation," "Fat," "Headaches."

CHOLESTEROL REGULATION

Controlling your cholesterol is absolutely essential to lowering your risk of atherosclerosis (cardiovascular disease), stroke, and heart attacks. Though medication may be required, wise nutrition is a very effective weapon for putting cholesterol in proper balance.

Basic Nutritional Therapy

In general, your goal should be to keep your total cholesterol under 200 milligrams per deciliter (of blood); your "good" cholesterol (HDL) above 50 mg/dl; your "bad" cholesterol lower than 130 mg/dl; and your ratio of total cholesterol to HDL cholesterol below 4.5 (if you are a man), or below 3.5 (if you are a woman). You can find your own cholesterol measurements from a blood test of your lipids (blood fats), which is available in almost every clinic and doctor's office.

A note on triglycerides: These lipids are connected to the cholesterol measurements and also pose an independent risk of heart disease. They should be lower than 125 and preferably below 100 for both men and women.

For a more precise listing of the meaning of cholesterol and tryglyceride measurements at different ages, see my *Controlling Cholesterol* (Bantam paperback, 1989, p. 53).

Special Food Sources, Strategies, and Facts

To keep your cholesterol at healthy levels, emphasize low-fat or no-fat foods such as skim milk, skim yogurt, vegetables, and fruits. Monounsaturated fats like olive oil have been linked to lower cholesterol levels. But saturated fats (found in whole milk, butter, or various meats) are the villain in the scenario; they trigger the production of excess cholesterol inside the body. (For a complete listing of these foods, along with menus, see my *Controlling Cholesterol*.)

It is important to eat enough foods with soluble fiber, such as oatmeal, beans, apples, and citrus fruits. Studies have shown that these foods are linked to lower levels of blood lipids, including cholesterol. (See the "Fiber, Insoluble" entry.)

Another good lipid-regulating food is deepwater fish. These fish have an abundance of omega-3 fatty acids, which many researchers feel have provided the Eskimos and other heavy fish eaters with added protection against cardiovascular disease. Fish in this category include: salmon, herring, mackerel, pompano, bass, cod, trout, tuna, and albacore.

There is also some evidence that alcohol can raise the "good" cholesterol in your blood, but it remains unclear whether the subcomponent of the good cholesterol affected by this drink is really protective against heart disease. (See "Alcohol.") As a result, I would not rely on alcohol to get your cholesterol ratio in balance.

In addition, some studies have shown that chocolate can raise "good" HDL cholesterol, probably because of the stearic acid in this sweet. (See "Chocolate.")

Finally, there is solid evidence that for many people, the "good" HDL cholesterol levels can be raised 10 percent or more through aerobic (endurance) exercise. Walking, jogging, or cycling three or four days a week, twenty to thirty minutes per session, will very likely do wonders to put your blood lipids in better balance.

Therapy Recommendations

Here are six basic nutritional recommendations about cholesterol that I believe you should follow:

1. Take off excess weight. Carrying even a few extra pounds can significantly increase your total cholesterol, including your "bad" cholesterol.

2. Reduce your intake of saturated fats. No more than 10 percent of the calories in your daily diet should come from saturated fats such as those found in meats, butter, or whole milk.

3. Increase your intake of monounsaturated fats, such as olive oil, rapeseed oil, or canola oil.

4. Limit your intake of cholesterol to no more than 300 milligrams per day. Keep the amount below 200 milligrams per day if you have a cholesterol problem or a family or personal history of heart disease.

5. Increase your intake of foods containing soluble fiber, such as oatmeal and citrus fruits. Several studies have shown that soluble-fiber foods can lower cholesterol levels.

6. Increase your intake of deepwater fish, such as salmon, tuna (white), herring, mackerel, and trout. These fish contain significant amounts of certain oils (the "omega-3 fatty acids," which include the all-important EPA acid or "eicosapentaenoic acid"). An abundance of these in the diet has been linked to lower levels of blood lipids, including triglycerides.

For more specific information on the amounts of cholesterol in various foods, and also on the way that soluble-fiber and omega-3 acids work, see my *Controlling Cholesterol*.

If you cannot bring your cholesterol into a healthy balance with these lifestyle changes, you may have to try a cholesterol-lowering medication. Products manufactured by several pharmaceutical companies have proved quite effective, with relatively few side effects for most people. See your physician for more information.

Cross-References

See "Alcohol," "Atherosclerosis," "Chocolate," "Fat," "Fiber, Insoluble," "Heart Disease."

CHROMIUM

Chromium is necessary for the proper functioning of insulin in the human body. Insulin plays a major role in metabolizing sugars and also is involved in the body's use of protein and fat. A borderline chromium deficiency may trigger adult-onset diabetes. *Caution:* Though a chromium deficiency may be the immediate trigger, it is *not* the underlying cause of diabetes, and so chromium supplements can't cure diabetes.

Satisfactory cholesterol and triglyceride levels have also been linked to adequate chromium levels in the body.

But other claims for chromium have been called into question. These include increased weight loss, muscle building, and greater longevity. Also, a dosage of 200 micrograms or more per day of chromium picolinate has been linked to iron deficiency.

Basic Nutritional Therapy

An estimated 50 percent of the American population has a marginal or serious chromium deficiency, according to Dr. Richard Anderson, a researcher for the Nutrition Center, a branch of the United States Department of Agriculture. (See *The New York Times*, December 6, 1995, p. B7.) Dr. Anderson believes that a safe and adequate daily intake of chromium is 50 to 200 micrograms. (But see the "downside" discussion below.)

A lack of chromium is particularly important if you are a diabetic or have a related blood-sugar or insulin problem. In such a case, it may be wise for you to go on chromium supplements—*but only under a qualified physician's supervision.*

Other possible uses of chromium may be more prevalent when additional scientific studies become available. For example, a few human and animal studies have resulted in lowered total cholesterol and raised levels of "good" HDL cholesterol. But this therapy is not part of the mainstream of medical treatment for cholesterol problems and is not recommended for most people.

The downside of chromium supplementation. Recent

studies have cast suspicion on the use of megadoses of chromium, particularly the popular supplement chromium picolinate, which is taken by millions of Americans. Findings by scientists at the Department of Chemistry, Dartmouth College, indicate that too much dietary chromium can accumulate in tissues to the point that damage occurs to chromosomes. This damage, which involves damage to the DNA, has been associated with the development of cancer. (See *Faseb Journal*, December 1995, pp. 1650-7.)

Reports presented at an N.I.H. workshop in Bethesda, Maryland, on supplements and exercise (June 3-4, 1996) warned that daily supplementation of 200 mcg or more of chromium picolinate may induce iron deficiencies.

How about chromium for athletes? Although chromium supplements are taken by many athletes to build muscle mass, there is strong disagreement as to whether the mineral is effective to help build muscles or promote a decrease in body fat. In one study reported in the *International Journal of Biosocial and Medical Research* (December 1989, pp. 163-180), football players increased their muscle mass after only two weeks of taking 1.6 milligrams of chromium picolinate. Also, their total body fat decreased from nearly 16 percent to about 12 percent.

Some athletes take as little as 600 micrograms (0.6 milligram) of chromium picolinate every day, considerably less than in the above study. But this is still three times the amount recommended by Dr. Anderson of the U.S. Department of Agriculture, and equivalent to the dose that produced chromosome damage to animals in the Dartmouth study.

Finally, not all of the scientific reports are positive. In 1994, a study was published in the *International Journal of Sports Medicine* by researchers at the University of Massachusetts at Amherst. They gave football players chromium supplements and found that the nutrients did not help build muscle or lose fat. There is no reason to think that chromium would increase muscle size or strength without a vigorous exercise program. (See *International Journal of Sports Nutrition*, 4:142, 1994.)

Special Food Sources, Strategies, and Facts

The best natural sources of chromium are whole grains, fruits, vegetables, brewer's yeast, wheat germ, liver, broccoli, prunes, nuts, cheese, and fortified cereals.

The estimated safe and adequate daily dietary intake, which is used when information is lacking to establish an RDA, is 50-200 micrograms daily.

Therapy Recommendations

Unless your physician directs otherwise, stick with foods to get your chromium. The benefits of unsupervised supplements are still far too uncertain and may result in damage to your health.

Cross-References

See "Cholesterol."

COENZYME Q10 (UBIQUINONE)

Coenzyme Q10, also known as "ubiquinone," behaves like a vitamin in the body by operating as a catalyst in various chemical interactions. It is essential to life and is found in every cell in our bodies. Coenzyme Q10 has attracted interest for its potential as an antioxidant, or a fighter against destructive free radicals in the body. But its primary job is to help convert the food we eat into energy. Various studies have suggested that this coenzyme could play a role in protecting the body against tissue damage from heart attacks, heart disease, retina deterioration, breast cancer, and a number of other diseases. But large, well-designed, double-blind scientific studies are hard to find.

Basic Nutritional Therapy

Because research into coenzyme Q10 is still at a relatively early stage, the use of supplements isn't advisable. But both human and animal studies have shown that this nutrient can provide a number of benefits, including the following (for more details on many of these conditions, see "Extra Scientific Information"):

- Protection against free radical damage to heart tissue when blood flows back into tissue that has been starved of blood after a heart attack
- Improvement of congestive heart failure
- Reduction of irregular heartbeats
- Improvement in hypertension, producing a decline in both systolic and diastolic blood pressure
- Protection of the heart against further damage (probably from free radicals) after heart surgery
- Regression of breast cancer
- Enhanced healing of periodontitis (inflammatory disease of the gums)
- Problems associated with deterioration of the retina

Because of these possible benefits, certain physicians may recommend coenzyme Q10 for specific treatment purposes. But the scientific investigation of Q10 is still at a preliminary stage, and so it's best to avoid taking any supplements unless you are directed to do so under medical supervision. Instead, focus on foods that are high in coenzyme Q10, including spinach, sardines, peanuts, and heart (beef). But keep in mind that some of these foods, such as beef heart, are very high in cholesterol and fat.

Extra Scientific Information

- Coenzyme Q10 is effective in limiting the severity of paralysis of the muscles of the eyes (ophthalmoplegia), according to research conducted in Australia in 1995. (See *Australian and New Zealand Journal of Ophthalmology*, August 1995, pp. 231-4.)
- Coenzyme Q10 has been used successfully against breast cancer, according to a 1995 report by Danish researchers. The patients took a daily oral dose of 390 milligrams of the coenzyme. (See *Biochemical and Biophysical Research Communications*, July 6, 1995, pp. 172-7. A related report can be found in *Molecular Aspects of Medicine*, 1994, 15 Supplement, pp. S231-40.)
- Coenzyme Q10 improved functioning of the mitochondria (energy cells) of the brain and also skeletal muscles in patients with retinitis pigmentosa (inflammation and atrophy of the retinal section of the eye). (See *Molecular Aspects of Medicine*, 1994, 15 Supplement, pp. S221-30.)
- Hypertensive patients were given daily doses of coenzyme Q10 (average dose: 225 milligrams), by physicians from the Institute for Biomedical Research at the University of Texas at Austin. The coenzyme was administered in addition to their regular drug regimen.

As a result of this treatment, the patients experienced significantly improved systolic and diastolic blood pressure measurements, and they were also able to cut back on their drug therapy. (See *Molecular Aspects of Medicine*, 1994, 15 Supplement, pp. S265-72.)

- More than 400 patients with various forms of cardiovascular disease were treated between 1985 and 1993 at the University of Texas Medical Branch,

Galveston, with an average dose of 242 milligrams of coenzyme Q10. The medical conditions included enlarged heart, hypertension, mitral valve prolapse, and heart valve disease.

Patients in each disease category showed significant improvement in heart function. Furthermore, no side effects from the treatment were noted, other than one transient case of nausea.

During the study, the overall medication requirements of the patients dropped considerably, with 43 percent eliminating between one and three of their drugs.

The researchers concluded that coenzyme Q10 is a safe and effective adjunctive treatment for a broad range of cardiovascular diseases. Furthermore, the relatively low price of the coenzyme eases the financial burden of multidrug therapy. (See *Molecular Aspects of Medicine*, 1994, 15 Supplement, pp. S165-75.)

- The heart responses of patients with chronic heart failure improved during exercise when they were given coenzyme Q10, according to research done in 1994 in Napoli, Italy. (See *Molecular Aspects of Medicine*, 1994, 15 Supplement, pp. S155-63.)
- Coenzyme Q10 was successfully used with adult periodontitis (inflammatory gum disease), both as a treatment by itself and also in combination with traditional nonsurgical periodontal therapy, Japanese researchers reported in 1994. (See *Molecular Aspects of Medicine*, 1994, 15 Supplement, S241-8.)
- Contrary to the above report, however, a review article in the March 15, 1995, issue of *British Dental Journal* (pp. 209-13) said that the claims of the benefits for coenzyme Q10 treatment in periodontal disease are overblown. In fact, there is some evidence

that coenzyme Q10 has no place in periodontal treatment.

- In animal studies conducted at the Medical College of Pennsylvania, treatment of the heart with coenzyme Q10 before ischemia (depriving the heart of blood) and reperfusion (putting blood back into the heart) improved heart function. One of the reasons for this improvement was that the coenzyme protected the heart tissue from oxidation damage, which typically results from an increase in free radicals. (See *Journal of Thoracic Cardiovascular Surgery*, February 1996, pp. 443-50.)
- Short-term oral doses of coenzyme Q10 (150 milligrams per day for two months) increased the circulation of the enzyme in middle-aged men and raised their perceived level of vigor. But the doses did not improve their performance in tests of aerobic capacity or forearm exercise metabolism. (See *International Journal of Sports Medicine*, October 1995, pp. 421-7.)
- In animal studies conducted at Kobe Gakuin University in Japan, coenzyme Q10 protected skeletal muscle cells against injuries from electrical stimulation. (See *Biochemical and Biophysical Research Communications*, November 22, 1995, pp. 1006-12.)
- Coenzyme Q10 may be able to protect vitamin E against oxidation from free radicals, according to lab studies at the University of Pittsburgh. (See *Archives of Biochemistry and Biophysics*, November 10, 1995, pp. 343-51.)
- When coenzyme Q10 is present in the "bad" LDL cholesterol in human blood, it can reduce the tendency of the LDL to become oxidized, reported researchers from the University of Ancona in Italy in 1995.

Note: Oxidation of LDL is a major factor in the development of atherosclerosis, or clogging of the arteries, which is the primary cause of heart attacks. (See *Procedures of the National Academy of Sciences*, U.S.A., September 26, 1995, pp. 9388-91.)

- Triathletes did not perform better on a treadmill, nor did cyclists cycle farther or faster, after taking 100 mg a day of coenzyme Q10 for four to eight weeks. (See *International Journal of Sports Medicine*, 2:272, 1992.)

Special Food Sources, Strategies, and Facts

Good food sources of coenzyme Q10 include: spinach, sardines, peanuts, and heart (beef).

Therapy Recommendations

Because research into coenzyme Q10 is still at a very early stage, at this point I cannot recommend that supplements be taken on a regular basis. Most people should obtain this nutrient through the food sources mentioned above.

On the other hand, studies have revealed that coenzyme Q10 *may* be helpful for those with a number of conditions, including hypertension, heart disease, special diseases of the retina, and even breast cancer. If you are in one of these health categories, your physician may recommend that you take coenzyme Q10 supplements. The literature indicates that a dosage of no more than 300 milligrams a day should not produce any side effects.

Cross-References

See "Heart Disease," "High Blood Pressure."

COMMON COLD

When lumped together with other self-limited upper respiratory problems like the flu, the common cold, which is caused by one or more of two hundred viruses, accounts for about half of all our illnesses.

Unfortunately, there is considerable truth to the old cliché about there being "no cure for the common cold." But that doesn't mean we have to give up all hope of protecting ourselves or finding some relief from this annoying threat to health. And one of our most powerful lines of defense is nutrition.

Basic Nutritional Therapy

The best strategy to avoid colds is to steer clear of people who have them, and to avoid touching your nose or face when you are in contact with cold sufferers. Because cold viruses come into the body through the nose, the first thing to do during cold season is to try to protect your nasal passages.

Many times, however, it's just not possible to avoid a cold-virus carrier. So, as a second line of defense, it's important to keep your immune system working at full blast. To this end, pay particular attention during cold season to managing the stress in your life effectively. Among other things, this means getting plenty of sleep and taking pains to avoid or at least respond well to pressure. Also, it's important not to overtrain in your athletic activities during the cold season. The more rundown you become from physical activity, the more you weaken your immune responses and your ability to fend off cold viruses and other diseases.

We all find ourselves in situations where we just can't avoid stress or manage it well. So, the final line of attack comes down to nutrition. An increasing body of evidence suggests that certain foods and supplements, especially those containing the antioxidant vitamins C, E, and beta-carotene, can contribute to your inner defenses against disease, including colds. (See "Extra Scientific Information.")

These antioxidants fight the free radicals (unstable oxygen molecules) generated in your body by job stress, overtraining, invading viruses, and other outside pressures. By mopping up the free radicals, the antioxidants help shore up your immune system.

In addition to antioxidants, some of my patients have found relief from cold symptoms by eating extra helpings of garlic and taking zinc throat lozenges (about 50 milligrams a day). Finally, increasing your intake of water and clear soups, such as chicken soup, will almost always mitigate symptoms and hasten recovery.

Extra Scientific Information

- Although one researcher concluded in 1975 that vitamin C is not beneficial in treating the common cold, later reviewers believe that vitamin C does significantly alleviate the symptoms of the common cold. (See *Journal of the American College of Nutrition*, April 1995, pp. 116-23.) The Finnish scientists in this review article calculated that taking 1 to 6 grams of vitamin C per day can decrease the duration of cold episodes by 21 percent.
- A "rhinovirus infection" (cold) tends to occur in these stages: (1) The virus enters into the body through the nose. (2) The virus is transmitted to the pharynx (throat). (3) The surface cells of the upper airways become infected. (4) The cold virus peaks within two days and persists for up to three weeks. (5) Infection is followed by inflammation of the tissues in the respiratory passages. (6) As we all know, the ongoing symptoms include sneezing, coughing,

and various aches and pains. (See *American Journal of Respiratory Critical Care and Medicine*, October 1995, pp. S36-9.)

- A study of nearly 900 workers in Oslo, Norway, confirmed that sharing office space with even one worker increases the risk of getting the common cold. Other risk factors include living with young children, having a history of hay fever, being female, and being under forty years of age. (See *European Journal of Epidemiology*, April 1995, pp. 213-6.)

- Day-care children under the age of two have an increased risk of getting the common cold, ear infection (acute otitis media), and pneumonia, according to a study at the University of Helsinki, Finland. (See *American Journal of Public Health*, August 1995, pp. 1109-12.)

Special Food Sources, Strategies, and Facts

Foods high in the antioxidant vitamin C are the most likely to provide nutritional defenses to the common cold viruses. These include all the citrus fruits, strawberries, cantaloupe, and vegetables such as broccoli, green peppers, and cauliflower. (See the "Vitamin C" entry and also Chapter 4.)

Therapy Recommendations

If you have a cold or feel one coming on, be sure that you are taking at least the minimum 1,000 milligrams of vitamin C per day, along with the other recommended antioxidants. The optimum amount of vitamin C just before and during a bout with a cold is even higher: 2,000 to 3,000 milligrams per day.

There is the possibility that adults who have been taking large doses of vitamin C for prolonged periods (e.g., 2,000 to 3,000 mg daily for several weeks) may tend to excrete more of the vitamin than usual. Sudden reduction in the dosage to 100 mg or less may cause symptoms of scurvy (such as anemia, weakness, or bleeding gums). Although this possibility is remote, to be safe when you discontinue use of the vitamin, I would advise reducing the amounts you take gradually.

To sum up: For adults consuming 1 to 2 grams of vitamin C per day, the risks are minimal. More than 2 grams per day may be a problem for some people. And those taking more than 8 grams per day should be aware of the distinct possibility of adverse side effects.

It's best to get as much vitamin C as possible through your food and then make up the remaining milligrams through supplements. (For more details on this therapy, see the recommendations under the "Vitamin C" entry and also in Chapter 4.)

Cross-References

See "Vitamin C," "Garlic," "Zinc," Chapter 4.

CONSTIPATION

Constipation is sometimes defined as the condition of having three or fewer bowel movements per week. But most experts feel that it's also important to include an additional factor: the ease or difficulty of having a movement.

If you regularly have problems eliminating waste, you have a constipation problem, even though you may have movements more than three times a week. (See *American Journal of Gastroenterology*, January 1996, pp. 26-32.)

Although some patients have to rely on over-the-counter laxatives or prescription medications, many find that they can overcome constipation exclusively through lifestyle changes and diet therapy. For more on this, see

"Basic Nutritional Therapy" and "Therapy Recommendations."

Basic Nutritional Therapy

The cornerstone of regular bowel movements, and the prime antidote to constipation, is fiber. (See the "Fiber, Insoluble" and "Fiber, Soluble" entries.) By taking in at least 20 to 35 grams of fiber per day, and preferably more, you will usually be able to overcome any problems with constipation. Some people may find they need to consume 40 or more grams per day, at least in the first stages of constipation treatment. But ultimately, for many people fiber is the answer.

Your emphasis should be on the *insoluble* type of fiber, which is found in vegetables, wheat, and cereals. Water-insoluble fibers accelerate the transit of the stool through the intestines. Soluble fiber, found in oats, citrus fruits, and the medication Metamucil®, will also promote bowel movements.

The main point in increasing the amount of fiber in your diet is to shorten the transit time for food to move through your intestinal tract. The faster the pace of your food, the less opportunity there is for it to become impacted. Also, shorter transit time has been associated with a decreased risk of colon (large intestine) cancer.

A second essential nutritional response to constipation is water. Taking in at least eight 8-ounce glasses per day, plus seven fruits and vegetables, will soften your stool considerably and make it much less likely that you will experience the pain of constipation. (See "Food Sources.")

Extra Scientific Information

- Constipation affects up to 20 percent of those sixty-five and older, according to the *Journal of Gerontological Nursing* (October 1995, pp. 21-30).

Older patients who receive a fiber supplement find they need to take a significantly lower number of laxatives each day than other patients. But because of possible side effects from fiber, such as gas or cramps, it's best to add fiber to the diets of these patients gradually, with close medical monitoring.

- A decline in frequency of bowel movements isn't an inevitable consequence of aging, said researchers at the Harvard Medical School. (See *Archives of Internal Medicine*, February 12, 1996, pp. 315-20.) They did find, however, that constipation and laxative use increase with advancing age, especially among women.
- Biofeedback failed to provide benefits for children who were suffering from constipation, according to a study at the University of Iowa Hospitals and Clinics. (See *Digest of Disease Science*, January 1996, pp. 65-71.)
- The causes of constipation in patients with advanced cancer are loss of appetite leading to reduced food intake, physical debilitation (including a sedentary lifestyle), and medications (especially opiate-derived pain relievers), according to researchers at St. Christopher's Hospice in London. (See *Cancer Survey*, 1994, pp. 137-46.)

Special Food Sources, Strategies, and Facts

If you have problems with constipation, weight your diet much more heavily in favor of wheat bran cereals, fruits, vegetables, and whole grain foods. An insoluble-fiber cereal in the morning is an essential part of nutritional treatment for constipation.

Also, increase your intake of water. I have suggested elsewhere that the average person can get by on fewer than eight 8-ounce glasses of water if he or she takes in plenty of fluids through fruits or fruit juices. But if you have a problem with constipation, I recommend that you consume at least four fruits and three vegetables per day, *and* that you drink eight 8-ounce glasses of water.

Finally, limit your intake of animal protein to 4 ounces per day, with 1 to 2 cups of dairy products. Avoid bananas, and other foods that tend to cause constipation.

Therapy Recommendations

Be sure to get regular aerobic (endurance) exercise each week. This means walking, jogging, or cycling at least three days a week, twenty to thirty minutes per session. This kind of body movement will help immensely in keeping your colon and digestive tract in shape.

Also, avoid over-the-counter laxatives unless your doctor has recommended them. If he has, check with him to work out a plan to cut back on the drugs while at the same time increasing your natural responses to constipation, including exercise and diet.

For details on specific types of foods that should help your constipation, see my remarks under "Food Sources."

Cross-References

See "Fiber, Insoluble," "Fiber, Soluble," "Water."

COPPER

Copper serves several important functions in the body, but its primary function is to serve as a constituent of enzymes. Its role in iron metabolism makes it a key factor in the synthesis of hemoglobin found in red blood cells. Copper also protects the bones against deterioration and osteoporosis, and it functions as a good antioxidant. Adequate copper supplies in the body have also been linked to lower levels of total cholesterol and higher amounts of "good" (HDL) cholesterol. Like iron, copper is needed in many of the reactions related to respiration and the release of energy.

Our body tissues contain an estimated 100 milligrams of this mineral, and daily intake requirements are rather small, about 1.5 to 3 milligrams per day. As a result, foods that contain copper should provide all that anyone needs. (See "Food Sources.")

Basic Nutritional Therapy

It's essential to maintain the right balance of copper in the blood and body tissues. Too little can result in a number of problems, including:

- Chorea, a disease of the nerves, often linked to rheumatic fever. It is marked by involuntary twitching of the muscles, face, and extremities.
- Spontaneous abortions and premature births.
- Anemia or insufficiency of red blood cells.
- Osteoporosis and other bone problems.
- High levels of cholesterol.

Too much copper in the body has been associated with increased susceptibility to infection, nausea, headaches, liver disease, leukemia, heart attacks, higher incidence of viral illnesses, and rheumatoid arthritis.

Because of the danger of taking in too much copper through supplements, and thus upsetting the delicate copper balance in the body, it's best to rely only on food and water for your daily supply. (See "Food Sources.")

Extra Scientific Information

- A study of forty-seven healthy five- to nine-year-old German children in 1995 revealed that their median intake of copper through the diet was in the lower range of the levels recommended by German nutrition agencies. (See *Annals of Nutritional Metabolism*, 1995, pp. 271-8.)

The children in the study took in these median amounts of nutrients every day: 1,578 calories of food, 46.5 grams of protein, 67.3 grams of fat, 174.7 grams of carbohydrates, 5.3 milligrams of zinc, and 0.7 milligrams of copper.

Note: The study found that the children's zinc intakes were also below the recommended nutritional levels.

- In a study conducted by King's College Hospital, London, British researchers reported that childhood cirrhosis of the liver is associated with high liver copper concentrations. The result is progressive liver disease, with high mortality rates. (See *Journal of Hepatology*, November 1995, pp. 538-43.)

Special Food Sources, Strategies, and Facts

Adequate daily intake of copper can be achieved through these foods: bran cereal, granola, toasted wheat germ (very high—0.7 milligram per cup), baking chocolate, buckwheat flour, whole wheat flour, wheat bran, brown rice, chocolate milk, whole milk, dried legumes, figs, dried peaches and pears, prunes, raisins, chuck beef, various beef steak cuts, beef liver (extremely high—3 milligrams for 4 ounces), boneless ham, various nuts (very high amounts in almonds, Brazil nuts, cashews, pecans, pistachios, walnuts), various seeds (especially pumpkin, sesame), duck, goose, pheasant, quail, clams, crab, lobster, oysters, snails, black bean soup, split pea soup, tomato soup, collards, kidney beans, lima beans, potatoes, soybean sprouts, vegetable juice cocktail, and yams.

Warning: High concentrations of copper in the body may result from the ingestion of copper from cookware and plumbing. As a result, it's wise to have the quality of your home drinking water tested periodically. To arrange for this procedure, check under the "Water" and "Laboratory Analysis" listings in your telephone Yellow Pages. Finally, do not cook with copperware.

Therapy Recommendations

Get your copper mainly from food sources, such as those listed above. Unless you are specifically directed to the contrary by a qualified physician, stay away from copper supplements.

Cross-References

See "Cholesterol."

CRAMPS

Muscle cramps can be caused by a variety of factors, some of which are nutritional. If you have experienced cramps during or after exercise, in the middle of the night following extended bed rest, or in other situations, you should consider examining your diet.

Basic Nutritional Therapy

If you experience cramps during or after an athletic workout or other intensive or unusual physical activity, several nutritional factors may be at work.

First of all, the heavy physical load may have caused you to perspire excessively and lose body salts, including potassium and salt (sodium chloride). The loss of these "electrolytes" can cause malfunctions in the muscles, with resulting cramps. The way to avoid this problem is to take in plenty of these minerals through your diet several hours before and after the activity. (See "Food Sources.")

Another possible cause of cramps after a strenuous

workout is the buildup of lactic acid in the muscles, representing the final stage in your body's exhaustion of its glycogen stores. A possible remedy is to eat a high-carbohydrate diet regularly, with at least 50 to 60 percent of daily calories coming from complex carbohydrates. Also, if you face a particularly demanding sports event, such as a distance race, you will want to try "carbohydrate loading." (See "Carbohydrates" entry, which includes a discussion of carbohydrate loading.)

Muscle cramps that occur at night are typically rapid, involuntary contractions of the leg muscles, usually the calf. They may last for a few seconds or for several hours. Often, some soreness will persist for the next 12 to 24 hours. An estimated 20 percent of the U.S. adult population has this problem, with most of the sufferers being in the elderly segment. The exact cause is unknown, but probably the condition results from inadequate blood supply, which may be associated with a lack of oxygen to the muscles.

Many over-the-counter products that claim to prevent leg cramps contain quinine and vitamin E. Even though physicians have been prescribing quinine as a muscle relaxant for decades, its side effects may outweigh the benefits, particularly in people over 60. (These negative effects include ringing in the ears, deafness, diarrhea, nausea, skin rashes, and visual disturbances.) In fact, the FDA may soon remove all over-the-counter drugs containing quinine.

In contrast, vitamin E, usually taken in one or two 400 IU capsules per day, has proven to be as effective as quinine and is relatively nontoxic when taken by mouth.

Another abnormality that causes leg cramping and pain with exercise is called "intermittent claudication." This condition, which is relieved by rest, is usually due to an insufficient blood supply to the legs. In some cases, vitamin E seems to provide relief.

Although vitamin E is virtually nontoxic, some people

have reported gastrointestinal problems, such as gas pains and cramps, when they consume more than 600 IUs per day. Also, high doses should not be used with blood thinners or anticoagulants.

Cramping may also result from taking diuretic drugs, such as those used for hypertension. These medications tend to reduce the body's fluid levels, with an accompanying loss of minerals, salts, and other nutrients. The proper response is to reduce the amount of your diuretic medication, switch medications, or increase your intake of fluids and electrolytes, particularly potassium.

Caution: Cramps may also arise from nonnutritional causes. If you are experiencing debilitating cramps, or if you find no improvement after a few days of trying a change in your nutritional program, be sure to see your physician.

Extra Scientific Information

- Cirrhosis of the liver may be accompanied by muscle cramps, probably because of the reduction of the effective circulating volume of the blood with this disease. (See *Hematology*, February 1996, pp. 264-73.)
- A 1995 study at East Carolina University School of Medicine in Greenville, North Carolina, noted that leg cramps in the elderly can be relieved through vitamin E, quinine sulfate, or stretching exercises. Though no treatment is effective for everyone, many patients find relief in one or more of them. (See *American Family Physician*, November 1, 1995, pp. 1794-8.)
- In another study, however, researchers at the Veterans Medical Center in Dayton, Ohio, cautioned that quinine, though effective for treating cramps, should be used in small doses, especially with the

elderly and with kidney patients. The dosages in this study involved taking 200 to 300 milligrams of quinine every night. But the researchers warned that quinine should be avoided completely by patients with liver disease. (See *Journal of Clinical Pharmacology*, June 1995, pp. 588-93.)

Special Food Sources, Strategies, and Facts

For a listing of food sources of complex carbohydrates, see the "Carbohydrates" entry. For example, important electrolytes like potassium can be obtained through such foods as orange juice, avocados, dried fruits, bananas, potatoes, nonfat yogurt, and sirloin steak.

For vitamin E food sources, see the "Vitamin E" entry. As you will see there, it is impossible to get all the vitamin E you need from your food. As a result, I recommend that the average person take vitamin E supplements in the range of 400 to 800 IUs per day. (For more details and specific recommendations for men and women in different age and activity categories, see chapter 4 and my *Antioxidant Revolution*, p. 127.)

Therapy Recommendations

To protect yourself from cramps, rely on your daily food program for at least 50 to 60 percent of your calories from complex carbohydrates. Increase that percentage if you participate in heavy sports activities. (See the "Carbohydrates" entry.)

Be sure to take your recommended daily level of vitamin E and other basic antioxidants. (See Chapter 4.)

Warning: If you suffer from severe muscle cramps, you may need quinine or large doses of vitamin E, but take these medications only under the supervision of your physician.

Cross-References

See "Vitamin B₆ (Pyridoxine)," "Carbohydrates," "Vitamin E," Chapter 4.

CREATINE SUPPLEMENTS

Creatine is a chemical found in the urine and also in muscle tissue. Operating as an enzyme in the muscle cells, it catalyzes phosphates into energy and plays an important role in muscle contraction. A naturally occurring compound found in considerable quantities in meat and fish, creatine should not be regarded as a drug.

Some athletes and bodybuilders use creatine supplements to increase their physical development and performance.

Basic Nutritional Therapy

Limited research has been done on this supplement, but some of the preliminary findings are intriguing.

In a study done at the Department of Physiology and Pharmacology, University of Nottingham Medical School, Queen's Medical Centre, United Kingdom, one group of bicyclists took placebos. Another group took 5-gram creatine supplements four times a day for five days. As part of the test, the participants engaged each day in three thirty-second bouts of maximal cycling.

The participants who took placebos showed no change in their athletic performance or in their body chemistry.

But the cyclists who took the creatine supplements significantly increased their "peak power output" in the first two bouts of exercise. However, they showed no improvement in the third exercise session. Also, the exercisers using creatine experienced lower accumulations of ammonia in their blood, a sign that their cellular energy production remained higher and more efficient than that of the athletes taking the placebos.

The researchers concluded that creatine ingestion can increase whole-body exercise performance during the initial two, but not a third, successive bouts of maximal exercise lasting thirty seconds. (See *European Journal of Applied Physiology*, 1994, pp. 268-76.)

Special Food Sources, Strategies, and Facts

Creatine is available commercially in both powder and tablet form. Its effectiveness seems to be in improving the performance of explosive exercise and increasing work output during repeated bouts of high-power physical activity. Also, it hastens recovery after exercise, thus allowing for longer and more intense training programs.

Studies demonstrating a beneficial effect of creatine have invariably involved the ingestion of 5 grams dissolved in 250 milliliters of a beverage four times a day, in the early morning, noon, afternoon, and evening (i.e., 20 grams per day for a period of five days). Muscle creatine stores are then maintained by ingesting only 2 grams daily. But creatine ingestion will not increase muscle stores beyond the normal natural limit.

Currently, creatine is not listed as a banned substance by any international sporting federation. Furthermore, because it is a naturally occurring constituent of a normal diet, it's unlikely to become a banned substance. (See *International Journal of Sports Nutrition*, 5:S100-10, 1995.)

But see "Therapy Recommendations" before you leap into this supplement.

Therapy Recommendations

Even though the above recommendations seem effective and safe, too little is known about the long-term effects of creatine use for me to recommend the supplements for general consumption. Also, in my own practice I've encountered at least one potential problem with this substance.

I have one patient who used creatine for several months quite effectively in his weight training program. He saw significant increases in both muscle mass and strength. But for some reason, perhaps creatine-related, he developed moderate to severe hypothyroidism (a decrease in the functioning of his thyroid gland). After he was taken off the creatine, his condition stabilized, but his body returned to normal only with thyroid supplementation.

Whether this was coincidental or a potential side effect of creatine is unknown. But before using these supplements, I strongly encourage you to get clearance from a physician who is a specialist in sports medicine. Also, have regular blood tests and physical examinations to be sure that your body's chemical balance remains stable and healthy.

Cross-References

See "Amino Acids," "Herbs."

CRUCIFEROUS VEGETABLES

Cruciferous vegetables, notably broccoli, brussels sprouts, cauliflower, and cabbage (the two "B's" and two "C's"), have been identified as strong anticancer weapons. They are also thought to be protective against other conditions including heart disease, diverticulitis, and constipation.

These vegetables, which are part of the *Brassica oleracea* species, were given the name "cruciferous" because their flowers grow in the form of an X-shaped Greek cross. Other edible plants in this group include tree kale and Portuguese cabbage.

Basic Nutritional Therapy

Eating cruciferous vegetables regularly, several times per week and preferably daily, has been connected to a lower incidence of a number of diseases, including: colon cancer, cancer of the esophagus, oral and pharyngeal (throat) cancers, thyroid cancer, and possibly cardiovascular disease.

A chemical component of cruciferous vegetables, indole-3-carbinol, has been identified as a key player in preventing breast cancer in women.

Also, the infants of breast-feeding mothers who eat cruciferous vegetables regularly have fewer problems with colic.

Extra Scientific Information

- There is evidence from University of Minnesota research that maternal intake of cruciferous vegetables during breast-feeding is associated with decline of colic symptoms in young infants. (See the *Journal of the American Dietary Association*, January 1996, pp. 46-8.)
- Increased levels of detoxification enzymes may explain the association between a high intake of cruciferous vegetables and a decreased risk of colorectal cancer, according to investigators from the University Hospital St. Radboud, Nijegen, the Netherlands. (See *Carcinogenesis*, September 1995, pp. 2125-8.) Participants in the study consumed a large amount of cruciferous vegetables: 300 grams per day of cooked brussels sprouts (about three cups).
- In animal studies conducted at the Department of Nutritional Sciences, University of Alabama, a chemical component of cruciferous vegetables, indole-3-carbinol, caused a significant decrease in

mammary tumors. (See *Anticancer Research*, May-June 1995, pp. 709-16.) The scientists concluded that indole-3-carbinol might be a good candidate for chemoprevention of breast cancer in women.

- In other animal studies at the University of South Florida, researchers determined that the natural antioxidant GSH, which has been associated with cancer-fighting properties, increased in the body after the consumption of diets high in cabbage or broccoli. (See *Nutrition and Cancer*, 1995, pp. 77-83.)
- Investigators at the National Institutes of Health reported a decreased risk of cancer of the esophagus with increased intake of raw fruits, vegetables, and fiber, including cruciferous vegetables. (See *Journal of the National Cancer Institute*, January 18, 1995, pp. 104-9.)
- Studies of indole-3-carbinol, an active chemical in cruciferous vegetables, suggest that eating more of these foods may help prevent breast cancer and other hormone-dependent cancers. (See *Steroids*, September 1994, pp. 523-7.)
- More than 1,000 patients with oral and pharyngeal (throat) cancers were studied by the National Cancer Center, National Institutes of Health, to see if there was a relationship between their diets and their disease. The researchers found that the patients' risk of having a second cancer was 40 to 60 percent lower among those with the highest intake of vegetables, including cruciferous vegetables. (See *Nutrition and Cancer*, 1994, pp. 223-32.)
- In a 1994 animal study conducted at the University of Mainz, Germany, all cruciferous vegetables, including broccoli and cauliflower, but with the exception of Chinese cabbage, were found to have

strong to moderate "antimutagenic" powers. In other words, they could protect genes from mutations characteristic of cancer growth. (See *Food Chemical Toxicology*, May 1994, pp. 443-59.)

- In a 1993 Swedish investigation into the risks of papillary thyroid cancer, a low intake of cruciferous vegetables was identified as an important risk factor, according to a report in *American Journal of Epidemiology*, October 1, 1993, pp. 482-91.

Special Food Sources, Strategies, and Facts

The basic cruciferous vegetables you should consider for your diet are broccoli, brussels sprouts, cauliflower, cabbage, turnips, and rutabagas. These complex carbohydrates not only have special cancer-fighting ingredients, such as indole-3-carbinol, they also contain an abundance of other nutrients that will help you fight disease and stay healthy. Here are just a few of the benefits of these power-packed foods:

- One cup of raw broccoli (about 90 grams) contains approximately 25 calories, with 2.5 grams from protein and 4.5 grams from complex carbohydrates. Also, this serving has more than 1,300 IUs of vitamin A, 85 milligrams of vitamin C, 65 micrograms of folic acid, 42 milligrams of calcium, 22 milligrams of magnesium, 290 milligrams of potassium, and various other vitamins, minerals, and amino acids.
- One cup of raw brussels sprouts has about 40 calories with 7.5 grams coming from carbohydrate and 3 grams from protein. In addition, this vegetable has approximately 800 IUs of vitamin A, 74 milligrams of vitamin C, 55 micrograms of folic acid, 35 milligrams of calcium, and 20 milligrams of magnesium.
- Cauliflower has considerably less vitamin A than

either broccoli or brussels sprouts, but more potassium than the other two.

- Common cabbage tends to have fewer nutrients per cup than the other cruciferous vegetables, probably because of the extra water it contains.

Because these vegetables are rather bitter, some people don't particularly like them. To increase your intake, try including them in salads with salad dressing, stir-fry them lightly, or use sauces to enhance the taste.

Therapy Recommendations

Eat at least one substantial helping (one cup) of cruciferous vegetables every day. Because of their greater overall nutritional value, I would recommend that you emphasize broccoli and brussels sprouts, with cauliflower in third place and cabbage in fourth.

Over the course of a week, try to vary your intake of the vegetables. For example, you might set aside three days for broccoli, two days for brussels sprouts, and one day for cauliflower. Or, you could try a mixture of these vegetables every day. By adding variety to your menu, you will be sure to get all the benefits of the cruciferous group.

Cross-References

See "Cancers," "Carbohydrates," "Vitamin C," "Fiber, Insoluble," "Fiber, Soluble," "Heart Disease."

VITAMIN D

Vitamin D is synthesized in the body through sunlight or is consumed with certain foods, like vitamin-fortified cereals, margarine, milk, egg yolks, and liver. The vitamin helps make phosphorus and calcium available in the blood, and contributes to the proper development and maintenance of bones and teeth.

A deficiency of vitamin D may result in rickets in children, a disease characterized by bone deformities that arise from a lack of vitamin D. In adults, the deficiency may lead to bone problems such as osteomalacia (softening of the bones through loss of calcium and protein). In addition, any failure of the body to synthesize vitamin D allows calcium to leave the bones, and that leads to the development of osteoporosis.

Basic Nutritional Therapy

Vitamin D is essential in the absorption of calcium by the body, and in this process helps prevent rickets in infants and bone deterioration in adults. In addition, this vitamin has been linked to reduced prostate cancer, improved parathyroid function, and lower blood pressure. Vitamin D may relieve symptoms of those suffering from Crohn's disease, an inflammatory disease of the lower intestine.

You need at least 400 IUs per day of vitamin D, and this dose can come through natural exposure of the hands, face, and arms to sunlight. About 10 to 15 minutes of exposure per day, four to five days a week, should provide more than enough for light-skinned people. Dark-skinned people require longer exposure (i.e., 30 minutes, four to five days a week). Foods fortified with vitamin D, such as certain cereals, milk, egg yolks, liver, butter, and fatty fish, can give you additional amounts of the vitamin.

Check the labels to see whether the foods are fortified and, if so, how much vitamin D they contain. One cup of most types of milk, for example, will provide 25 percent of your daily vitamin D needs, or about 100 IUs.

Vitamin D supplements are not needed unless you are unable to go outdoors, or your physician directs otherwise. This vitamin is quite powerful and in excessive doses can produce toxic effects, with a variety of health problems.

Symptoms may start with apathy, headaches, fatigue, loss of appetite, and excessive thirst, and progress to serious damage to the kidneys, lungs, heart, and bones.

Extra Scientific Information

- In a study of more than 300 healthy women ages seventy and older, low blood levels of vitamin D were associated with "secondary hyperparathyroidism," a disease characterized by excessive secretions of the parathyroid glands, resulting in loss of calcium from the bones, kidney stones, and other problems. Also, the women experienced a significant loss of bone mass. (See *Journal of Bone and Mineral Research*, August 1995, pp. 1177-84.)
- Researchers at the University Hospital, Uppsala, Sweden, reported that vitamin D might be used to control rejection of organ transplants by the body. (See *Transplant Immunology*, September 1995, pp. 245-50.)
- Vitamin D supplementation did *not* bring about a decrease in hip fractures in elderly Dutch patients in a 1996 study at the Vrije Universiteit, Amsterdam, the Netherlands. (See *Annals of Internal Medicine*, February 15, 1996, pp. 400-6.)
- Higher blood serum levels of vitamin D may slow the progression of prostate cancer in both black and white men, especially after age fifty-seven, according to scientists at Duke University. (See *Cancer Epidemiology and Biomarkers Preview*, September 1995, pp. 655-9.)
- Serum levels of vitamin D are inversely related to blood pressure levels, according to a report from the Department of Internal Medicine, University Hospital, Uppsala, Sweden. The higher the vitamin D levels in the blood, the lower the blood pressure.

(See *American Journal of Hypertension*, September 1995, pp. 894-901.)

- In animal studies at Louisiana State University, consumption by mothers of a low-vitamin D diet resulted in a general but significant slowing of cardiac development of the unborn offspring. Whether this occurs in humans is unknown. (See *Journal of Molecular and Cellular Cardiology*, June 1995, pp. 1245-50.)

- Patients with Crohn's disease, an inflammation of the lower intestine, must consume a diet high in vitamin D or rely on vitamin D supplementation to overcome the negative effects of low sun exposure on their bone mineral density. The researchers in this 1995 study noted that patients with this disease tend to have a low amount of sun exposure in the summer months. (See *Wien Klin Wochenschr*, 1995, pp. 578-81.)

Special Food Sources, Strategies, and Facts

The best sources of vitamin D are sunlight and foods like fortified milk, margarine, cereals, butter, egg yolks, liver, fatty fish, fish oils, and certain ocean fish like tuna and halibut.

Therapy Recommendations

You should get the necessary amount of vitamin D from exposure to sunlight if you spend at least 10-15 minutes a day, four or five days a week. But take care not to *over*expose your skin. Remember the dangers of skin cancer.

Also, include in your diet the foods mentioned under "Food Sources."

You should take supplements only if your physician recommends you to do so.

Cross-References

See "Calcium."

DERMATITIS AND OTHER SKIN PROBLEMS

Dermatitis, an inflammation of the skin that may be accompanied by flaking, scaliness, or itching, can be caused by allergic reactions to certain foods. Also, manipulation of nutrition by either dietary restriction or supplementation can help with skin conditions such as skin cancer, wound healing, atopic (allergic) dermatitis, psoriasis, and problems related to herpes.

Basic Nutritional Therapy

Seborrheic dermatitis is a common condition that appears as simple dandruff. The inflammation may also be found on the face, the chest, or the creases of the arms, legs, or groin.

The most common sufferers of seborrheic dermatitis are infants and adults between the ages of thirty and sixty. Generally, the best treatment is a topical application of certain creams or preparations, including those made up of steroids, selenium, coal tar, or zinc. (See *American Family Physician*, July 1995, pp. 149-55, 159-60.)

Other types of dermatitis may be triggered by sensitivity to grains such as wheat or oats, by a zinc deficiency, by soybeans, or even by cobalt found in fortified beer.

One of the most common treatments is to avoid the foods or nutrients that cause dermatitis. Also, some patients have found their symptoms disappear after they take fish oil or corn oil preparations.

Of course, it may also be necessary to rely on an anti-allergy medication prescribed by your doctor.

Extra Scientific Information

- Finnish children developed dermatitis after inhaling cereal particles or ingesting certain cereals containing wheat or oats, according to research at the Helsinki University Central Hospital in 1995. (See *Clinical Experiments in Allergy*, November 1995, pp. 1100-7.) The children in this study also showed sensitivity to rice, corn, millet, and buckwheat.
- Dutch children with a zinc deficiency developed dermatitis. Other symptoms common among these children were diarrhea, recurring infections, and growth retardation. (See *Biological Trace Elements Research*, August-September 1995, pp. 211-25.)
- Heavy consumers of cobalt-fortified beer have experienced cardiomyopathy or heart disease. It's also known that cobalt is able to cause allergic dermatitis, rhinitis, and asthma. (See *Science of the Total Environment*, June 30, 1994, pp. 1-6.)
- Patients with allergic (atopic) dermatitis were given fish oil or corn oil in a 1994 study conducted over a four-month period at the University of Oslo, Norway.

One group of patients received 6 grams per day of fish oil, and a second group got a comparable amount of corn oil. The dermatitis of those in the fish oil group improved by 30 percent, and the condition of those in the corn oil group improved by 24 percent. (See *British Journal of Dermatology*, June 1994, pp. 747-64.)

Special Food Sources, Strategies, and Facts

To determine the cause of dermatitis, you should be tested by your personal physician, a dermatologist, or an allergy specialist. If the cause of your problem is nutrition related, you will probably have to go on an "elimination diet." (See the "Allergies" entry.)

Therapy Recommendations

Fish oil containing the omega-3 fatty acids and also Chinese herbal tea have been effective in treating atopic (allergic) dermatitis.

Studies have also shown that psoriasis can be responsive to vitamin A and D treatments. Although fish oil has not been effective in treating psoriasis, there is a strikingly low incidence of psoriasis in Greenland Eskimos.

Before you plunge into one of these treatments for your skin problems, however, take note of the implications if you are concerned about your cardiovascular risk:

Fish oil with omega-3 fatty acids has proven to have beneficial effects on blood fats and cholesterol profiles of patients. But synthetic vitamin A can cause an elevation in the blood triglycerides, an increase in the "bad" LDL cholesterol, and a decrease in the "good" HDL cholesterol. So with prolonged vitamin A therapy, there could be an increase of atherosclerosis.

Vitamin A and its derivatives (the "retinoids") have been used more effectively in treating acne (Retin-A® is one medication) than skin cancers. In one study, retinoid treatment of skin cancers found that 51 of 57 patients responded positively, either partially or completely, to oral retinoids. But the high doses of oral retinoids used in this and comparable studies have caused significant side effects. (See the "Vitamin A" entry for a list of possible side effects.)

Vitamin A and fish oil are not the only possibilities for your skin problems. Topical and oral selenium, for instance, can provide protection against ultraviolet induced sunburn, tanning, and skin cancer. Topical vitamin C also has been shown to be protective against light, and vitamin C can act locally on the skin as an antioxidant.

Nutritional deficiencies may also retard wound healing. These include low levels of protein, vitamin A, vitamin C, vitamin K, and zinc. It's been known for centuries that a deficiency of vitamin C can impair wound healing, but the power of vitamin A supplementation to heal skin damage has been known only since the 1940s.

Supplementation may be of value in some patients, even if they don't show signs of being nutritionally depleted. But the benefits of oral zinc supplementation in patients who are not zinc-deficient have yet to be established.

More on skin cancer: Several studies have evaluated the use of beta-carotene, a precursor of vitamin A, in treating non-melanoma skin cancers (i.e., the least serious form of skin cancer). In laboratory animals, treatment with oral beta-carotene has inhibited the development of skin cancers induced by chemicals or ultraviolet light. In one study of 1,805 patients with recently diagnosed skin cancers, people taking 50 mg of oral beta-carotene (approximately 80,000 IU) daily for five years showed no differences from a placebo group. Another study indicated that 100 mg of beta-carotene (approximately 160,000 IU) daily is necessary to protect patients from sun-induced cancers.

Additional study of dietary manipulation and the effect of nutritional supplementation on the skin and skin diseases is necessary. But as the above discussion indicates, there are certainly some promising early results in this field. (See *Journal of the American Academy of Dermatology*, 1993, pp. 447-61.)

Cross-References

See "Vitamin A," "Allergies," "Cancers," "Selenium," "Wounds, Healing," "Zinc."

DHEA

DHEA, the popular abbreviation for "dehydroepiandrosterone," is a hormone that was first discovered in 1934. Although scientists have been puzzling over its significance for years, it has been promoted as an antiaging drug, and also as a means of improving immunity, lowering cholesterol, promoting growth gains in muscle and bone, and improving cardiovascular function. DHEA has also been considered as a treatment for AIDS and lupus, though there is no proven benefit as yet in these areas.

Fully formed DHEA is not found in plants, though a natural precursor is present in yam extracts (diosogenin or discorea). This precursor may be used by the body to make DHEA, but in older people, the precursor does not seem to be converted to DHEA. (See *Journal of Immunology*, 150:2219-30, 1993.)

A prescription is needed for fully formed DHEA, but the FDA has not approved it yet for treatment of any conditions. Until 1986, it was a nonprescription drug, but it was reclassified at that point by the FDA since its long-term risks are unknown.

Basic Nutritional Therapy

DHEA supplementation may improve or restore immunity, according to a study published in the *American Journal of Obstetrics and Gynecology* in 1993 (pp. 1536-9). In this investigation, 50 milligrams of DHEA per day for three weeks increased the natural killer cells, the body's main defense against cancer.

Other possible uses of DHEA involve restoring the immune function or at least slowing the malfunctions that occur with leukemia. Also, the medication has been used in treatment of AIDS, even though no definitive positive results have been recorded. (See *Experiments, Opinions and Investigations with Drugs*, 4:147-54, 1995.)

On the aging issue, decreased levels of DHEA in the body have been correlated directly with increased mortality (deaths) in aged men. Most likely, the reason was that the immune system begins to become unbalanced with age, with the loss of some functions and an increase in others. These changes may account for a rise in arthritis and leukemia among the elderly. A normalization of this immune response has been seen in aged mice in response to DHEA supplementation. (See *Journal of Immunology*, 150:2219-30, 1993.)

There are a number of other possible dangers of DHEA that bear watching. Using rats as experimental animals, scientists found that fourteen out of sixteen of those on DHEA developed liver cancer. That doesn't mean the same thing would happen in humans, but if such a response did occur in humans, the FDA would ban it. (See *University of California Wellness Letter*, January 1996.)

Also, the effects of DHEA replacement have not been studied beyond six months. Therefore, we don't know the benefits or the hazards of long-term use. The implications for improving well-being, particularly in the aged, have involved only limited study. (See *Journal of the American Medical Association*, 265:912, 1997.)

Extra Scientific Information

Whether the effects of DHEA come from the hormone itself or from sex hormones and other steroids that the body produces is unknown. We are not even sure which organs the substance affects.

Originally, DHEA was sold in health food stores as a means of losing weight. But in 1985, the FDA forced manufacturers to stop promoting it for weight loss since it had never been reviewed for either safety or effectiveness.

Because DHEA is a naturally occurring substance, it can't be patented. Consequently, it is unlikely that any drug company will spend millions of dollars on clinical trials to determine its effectiveness, as required by the FDA. In the meantime, drug companies are testing synthetic forms of DHEA, including extracts from yams, as possible treatment for AIDS and lupus erythematosus. (See *University of California Wellness Letter*, January 1996.)

Special Food Sources, Strategies, and Facts

The only natural food source of DHEA is its precursor, the extract of wild yams (diosogenin or discorea). Otherwise, a prescription is required to obtain DHEA.

Therapy Recommendations

At present, I am not convinced that DHEA is either effective or safe, and so I am not prescribing it for my patients. But I have no objections to their eating yams or using wild yam cream for its phytoestrogen effect. (See the "Hormones" entry, specifically the discussion on hormone replacement therapy, or HRT.)

Cross-References

See "Hormones."

DIARRHEA

Many nonnutritional factors may contribute to diarrhea, including: the ingestion of certain antibiotics, abuse of enemas or laxatives, poisoning by iron or insecticides, viruses, bacteria, parasites, cancer, and other diseases such as diverticulitis. (See "Cancers," "Diverticulitis, Diverticulosis.") But there are also a number of possible nutritional causes of diarrhea.

Basic Nutritional Therapy

Some of the nutritional triggers for diarrhea include:

- Milk and dairy products. Those with a lactose (milk sugar) intolerance, which comes from low levels of the lactase enzyme, may experience diarrhea, cramps, or gas after consuming dairy foods. (See "Calcium.") If you have this problem, see your physician for specific recommendations and medications.
- Folate (folic acid) deficiency. To correct this problem, eat more foods with folic acid, including dark green leafy vegetables, organ meats, brewer's yeast, and whole grain products. In addition, take folic acid supplements of at least 400 micrograms per day. (See the "Folic Acid" entry and also Chapters 2 and 3.)
- Large doses of vitamin C. Some people have reported that taking megadoses of vitamin C supplements, in excess of about 2,000 milligrams per day, produces diarrhea.

Note: Most patients I deal with who take large doses of vitamin C do not report any problem with diarrhea.

- Excessive amounts of fiber. Most people seem to have a gastrointestinal threshold for bran cereals, fruits, vegetables, and other high-fiber foods. Their stools remain solid but soft up to a point; then when they take in too much fiber, diarrhea results.

You should eat at least five to seven servings of fruits and vegetables each day, and you should also include a high-fiber cereal on your breakfast table every morning. But you will find it necessary to balance your fiber with foods that tend to make the stool more solid, such as dairy products (for those without lactose intolerance), or bananas.

- Zinc deficiency. (See "Extra Scientific Information.")
- Apple juice. (See "Extra Scientific Information.")
- Problems with maternal breast milk. (See "Extra Scientific Information.")
- Sorbitol. This natural sweetener is used in many medications and supplements, as well as in "sugar-free" candies and gums.

Sorbitol can cause abdominal cramping and diarrhea. Usually, it takes about 50 grams to cause diarrhea, but at times, as little as 10 grams will trigger a problem. That's the amount in only three to five "sugar-free" mints.

Sorbitol is also found in vitamins and various medications. Because it's not an "active" ingredient, the Food and Drug Administration doesn't require it to be listed separately on labels.

Extra Scientific Information

- Researchers at the Department of Pediatrics, Drechtsteden Hospital Jacobus, Zwijndrecht, the Netherlands, conducted a study in 1995 of children with zinc deficiencies. They found that those with some zinc deficiency experienced diarrhea, recurrent infections, and, in the worst cases, growth retardation. The scientists' conclusion: Children with these deficiencies should be treated with supplements. (See *Biological Trace Elements Research*, August-September 1995, pp. 211-25.)
- Patients with chronic intestinal disease, including diarrhea, should be evaluated for likely deficiencies and imbalances of essential fatty acids (EFAs), according to a 1996 report from the Boston University Medical Center Hospital. Furthermore, these patients should be treated with substantial amounts of supplements rich in EFAs, including

vegetable and fish oils, or intravenous lipids if necessary. (See *Metabolism*, January 1996, pp. 12-23.)

- A fifty-one-year-old patient's poor diet may have contributed to her deficiency of folate (folic acid) and resulting diarrhea, severe weight loss, and other symptoms that required a long hospital stay. (See *Nutrition in Clinical Practice*, December 1994, pp. 247-50.)

- Chronic diarrhea may be caused by dietary factors, including apple juice, Dutch researchers reported in 1995. In the ten children who were studied, the investigators found that clear, processed apple juice promoted diarrhea significantly, while cloudy apple juice did not. The researchers believed that the presence of fructose and the processing method used in the clear juice may have resulted in diarrhea. (See *Archives of Disease in Children*, August 1995, pp. 126-30.)

- The breast milk of mothers infected with H. pylori bacteria (which is associated with chronic gastritis and duodenal ulcers) caused diarrhea in nursing infants, according to research at the University of Glasgow, Yorkhill Hospitals, Scotland. (See *Transcripts of the Royal Society Tropical Medical Hygiene*, July-August 1995, pp. 347-50.)

Special Food Sources, Strategies, and Facts

See "Basic Nutritional Therapy" and "Extra Scientific Information."

Therapy Recommendations

Chronic or recurrent diarrhea should always be treated by a physician. Short-term bowel problems, however, can often be managed at home.

To control short-term diarrhea that you think arises

from nutritional causes, the first step is to eliminate foods or additives (such as sorbitol) that may be causing the problem. (See "Basic Nutritional Therapy" above.) Many of my patients have identified their lactose intolerance tendencies just by seeing their symptoms disappear after they cut down on milk or other dairy products. But, if you take this route, be sure that you get adequate calcium through other sources. (See "Calcium.")

If you have no success after eliminating one or two suspected foods, you should consult your doctor. You may have to add extra nutrients to your diet to control the problem. This step is more complicated and usually requires the advice of a registered dietitian or a nutritionally trained physician.

Cross-References

See "Vitamin C," "Calcium," "Cancers," "Diverticulitis, Diverticulosis," "Fiber, Insoluble," "Fiber, Soluble," "Folic Acid, Folate," "Water," "Zinc," Chapters 2 and 3.

DIVERTICULITIS, DIVERTICULOSIS

Diverticulosis is a condition of the colon, or large intestine, which involves the development of sacs or pouches that extend out from the walls of the colon into the surrounding body cavities. An estimated 10 percent of people over age forty, and nearly one-half of people over age sixty, have some form of diverticulosis.

When food or other particles get stuck in these sacs, inflammation and infection may result and lead to the condition known as diverticulitis. This disease is signaled by severe lower abdominal pains and fever. The final result of diverticulitis may be the highly dangerous, potentially deadly condition known as peritonitis, which occurs when the sacs burst and the abdominal lining becomes infected.

Fortunately, good nutrition can help you prevent this disease, or lessen its effects if you already have it.

Basic Nutritional Therapy

The basic nutritional approach to prevent or treat diverticulitis is to eat plenty of fiber. Everyone should be taking in at least 20 to 35 grams of fiber per day, an amount that should be adequate to prevent most cases of diverticulosis from degenerating into diverticulitis. (See "Food Sources.")

The best nutritional response to diverticulitis is insoluble fiber, which is found in wheat bran, vegetables, and other foods containing plenty of cellulose (such as broccoli). Insoluble fiber is the best kind of food to increase the transit time and efficient passage of food through your intestinal tract. The faster the food moves through your colon, the less likely it is that infection and inflammation will develop.

It is also wise to round out your fiber diet with foods containing soluble fiber, which is found in oats, potatoes, beans, peas, lentils, strawberries, and apples. This type of fiber is not quite as efficient as the insoluble type in increasing bowel transit time, but it's still much more effective at this job than many other foods. (See "Fiber, Insoluble," and "Fiber, Soluble.")

Special Food Sources, Strategies, and Facts

Refer to the foods mentioned above in "Basic Nutritional Therapy," and also check the entries on "Fiber, Insoluble," and "Fiber Soluble."

The best preventive measure against diverticulitis is to consume at least 20 to 35 grams of fiber per day, with an emphasis on insoluble fiber.

To get this much in one day, you could eat one pear (4 grams of fiber), one-half cup of bran cereal (15 grams), one whole apple (4 grams), one-half cup of cooked broccoli (2.5 grams), one-half cup of cooked navy beans (8 grams), and one cup of cooked whole wheat spaghetti (5 grams). That would be 38.5 grams of fiber in one day, with approximately an equal mix of soluble and insoluble fiber.

Therapy Recommendations

A fiber-rich diet containing 20 to 35 grams a day of fiber may prevent diverticula (pouches that grow out from the intestines) from forming. This sort of diet can also prevent constipation and subsequent irritation of existing pouches. (See the "Food Sources" above.)

Some doctors recommend avoiding irritating foods like popcorn, nuts, and seeds, which may lodge in the diverticula and cause an infection (diverticulitis).

Therapy for acute diverticulitis usually includes bed rest, antibiotics, and a clear liquid diet. At times, hospitalization is necessary. Following an acute attack, a very low-fiber diet is recommended until the bowels heal. Once the acute symptoms subside, the high-fiber diet may be used. Surgery occasionally is required, particularly with complications.

Cross-References

See "Constipation," "Fiber, Insoluble," "Fiber, Soluble."

VITAMIN E

Vitamin E is an anticoagulant (blood thinner) as well as a powerful antioxidant that fights the destructive effects of free radicals (unstable oxygen molecules) in the body.

It has been linked to a reduced risk of cardiovascular disease because of its ability to neutralize the oxidation of "bad" LDL cholesterol. The oxidation of LDL is a primary factor in the buildup of plaque in the blood vessels, which leads to atherosclerosis and heart attacks.

An increasing body of evidence, including research we are doing at the Cooper Institute for Aerobics Research, indicates that vitamin E can protect both elite athletes and those engaging in moderate exercise (the equivalent of walking vigorously or jogging twenty to thirty minutes a day, three to four days a week) from damage to DNA in the body's cells. Such damage has been associated with a higher incidence of cancer and other diseases. In other studies, vitamin E has been linked to a lower risk of cancer and cataracts, and also increased immunity.

Basic Nutritional Therapy

The most recent studies on vitamin E show that the full health benefits flow from a daily intake of 400 to 1,200 IUs per day. The only way to do this is to rely on a natural vitamin E supplement.

I recommend that every adult take at least 400 IUs per day through supplements (look for *natural* vitamin E, indicated by the term "d-alpha tocopherol" on the bottle label). Those who weigh more than 200 pounds or who are active athletes should take closer to 1,200 IU. (For my specific recommendations for men, women, children, and those in various activity categories, see Chapter 3.)

Unfortunately, it's next to impossible to get an adequate daily dose of vitamin E through the diet. The richest sources have relatively low amounts of the vitamin; also, the best foods are high-calorie, high-fat oils and nuts. Examples are wheat germ oil, soybean oil, almonds, and hazelnuts.

Here's an illustration of the problem of relying exclusively on foods for your vitamin E. One tablespoon of wheat germ oil has only about 30 to 35 IUs of vitamin E (plus 120 calories); one cup of hazelnuts has about 30 IUs (plus more

than 800 calories); and one cup of almonds has about 20
IUs (plus more than 800 calories). You can see that it would
be very difficult to reach 400 IUs per day by eating such
foods without putting on many extra pounds.

Extra Scientific Information

- Vitamin E succinate (a common derivative of vitamin E used in supplements) inhibits the proliferation of prostate cancer cells, according to a 1995
  study at the Division of Nutritional Sciences,
  University of Texas at Austin. (See *Nutrition and
  Cancer*, 1995, pp. 161-9.)
- Animal studies at the University of Munich,
  Germany, show that vitamin E in the diet can reduce
  the extent of "reperfusion injury" after body tissue is
  deprived of blood (ischemia). This type of injury is
  common after a heart attack, when the heart is first
  deprived of blood and then blood flows back into the
  starved tissue through collateral blood vessels. (See
  Free Radical Biology and Medicine, December 1995,
  pp. 919-26.)
- Antioxidants such as vitamin E protect "bad" LDL
  cholesterol from oxidation, which is a major step in
  the buildup of plaque and atherosclerosis, according
  to researchers at the University of Zurich,
  Switzerland. The investigators who studied patients
  with cystic fibrosis believe that LDL resistance to
  oxidation is impaired in vitamin E-deficient
  patients, but can be normalized within two months
  when the vitamin is given in sufficient amounts.
  They gave their patients 400 IUs of vitamin E daily
  for the two-month period. (See *Free Radical Biology
  and Medicine*, December 1995, pp. 725-33.)
- Vitamin E and vitamin A worked together effectively,
  with a "synergistic" action, to reduce oxidation of

lipids, according to a study done at the Universita di Palermo, Italy. (See *Archives of Biochemistry and Biophysics*, February 1, 1996, pp. 57-63.) The researchers think that vitamin E helped limit the oxidation of vitamin A, and thus strongly promoted the effectiveness of the vitamin A. Also, the combination therapy helped slow down the destruction of the vitamin E.

• In cystic fibrosis, there may be a deficiency of vitamin E that may accelerate oxidation of "bad" LDL cholesterol, promote atherosclerosis, and also have an adverse effect on the lungs. Vitamin E is recommended as a part of the therapeutic regimen for these patients. (See *Free Radical Biology and Medicine*, 1995, pp. 725-33.)

Special Food Sources, Strategies, and Facts

As mentioned above, the best type of vitamin E is the natural variety called "d-alpha tocopherol." (Synthetic vitamin E has an "L" in the technical name: "dl-alpha tocopherol.")

For more on this vitamin, see the discussion above under "Basic Nutritional Therapy." Also, for up-to-date details on vitamin E, refer to Chapter 4.

Therapy Recommendations

See "Basic Nutritional Therapy" above, Chapter 4, and page 127 of *Antioxidant Revolution* for my specific recommendations on vitamin E and the other antioxidants.

Cross-References

See "Vitamin A," "Vitamin C," Chapter 4.

ELECTROLYTES

Electrolytes are salts that dissolve in water, and, in the form of solutions, can conduct electricity. They play an active role in body metabolism and functioning. They include such substances as potassium, sodium, and the chlorides.

An electrolyte deficiency or imbalance may develop as a result of illness, vomiting, diarrhea, excessive perspiration, inadequate diet or fluid intake, blood pressure medications, or other drugs. When that happens, the patient will begin to display certain telltale symptoms, such as unusual fatigue, weakness, disorientation, dizziness, or even paralysis.

If a serious electrolyte deficiency isn't treated fairly quickly, there can be serious health consequences, including death. Intravenous fluids may have to be given to patients who have lost too much water or body salts.

Basic Nutritional Therapy

Drink eight 8-ounce glasses of water per day, or the equivalent in natural fruit juices or juicy fruits. Also, be sure to eat plenty of fruits and vegetables, which contain many of the electrolytes your body needs to maintain a good chemical balance. (See "Carbohydrates.")

If you are exercising or working hard and are perspiring a great deal, drink extra water, and also consider using an electrolyte-fortified sports drink. For maximum effect, some of these special electrolyte drinks containing potassium and other important body salts should be diluted by one-half with water.

Caution: If you have hypertension, a kidney problem, or any other medical condition that might respond negatively to increasing your intake of salts, check with your physician first. (See "Extra Scientific Information" below.)

Extra Scientific Information

- In a 1995 study conducted at the Food Safety Control and Inspection Institute, Tianjin, People's Republic of China, researchers concluded that factors contributing to high blood pressure in Tianjin were related to age, body mass index, high sodium intake, and a high sodium-to-potassium ratio. (See *Journal of Hypertension*, January 1995, pp. 49-56.)
- Researchers at Loughborough University of Technology in Britain examined the effects on endurance capacity during exercise of drinking a carbohydrate-electrolyte solution.

The trained athletes participating in the study performed two exercise trials, seven days apart. During these trials, they engaged in seventy-five-minute sessions, divided into five fifteen-minute periods of sprinting, jogging, and walking.

Half of the exercisers were given the electrolyte solution, and half a placebo. They were all instructed to take their drinks immediately prior to exercise and every fifteen minutes thereafter.

The results showed that drinking a carbohydrate-electrolyte solution improves endurance-running capacity during prolonged intermittent exercise. (See *Journal of Sports Science*, August 1995, pp. 283-90.)

- A review of twenty-nine studies investigating the effects of sodium bicarbonate on anaerobic exercise performance revealed that overall performance was enhanced by the supplement. Anaerobic exercise involves events like sprints, which are characterized by high-intensity exercise, causing the body to use up more oxygen than it takes in. In contrast, aerobic or endurance exercise is characterized by activities that balance the output and intake of oxygen. (See

International Journal of Sports Nutrition, March 1993, pp. 2-28.)

Special Food Sources, Strategies, and Facts
See "Basic Nutritional Therapy."

Therapy Recommendations
See my recommendations under "Basic Nutritional Therapy."

Cross-References
See "Electrolytes," "Salt," "Water."

EYE COMPLAINTS

An increasing number of nutrition-based therapies are able to prevent or treat various eye problems. In particular, the evidence is strong for using your diet to fight cataracts and age-related macular degeneration (AMD).

Basic Nutritional Therapy
The main dietary antioxidants—vitamin E, vitamin C, and beta-carotene—have been linked to a reduced risk of cataracts. (See "Vitamin A," "Vitamin C," "Cataracts.")

A decreased incidence of age-related macular degeneration (AMD) is associated with the intake of the carotenoids lutein and zeaxanthin, which are present in dark, leafy greens such as collards and spinach. This disease is the major cause of blindness in Americans over sixty-five years old, or 25 percent of the American population. (See discussion under the "Vitamin A" entry.)

It has been suggested that many eye-related diseases are caused or aggravated by the presence of free radicals, the unstable oxygen molecules in the body that can damage cells and tissue. Antioxidants help to counter the destructive work of the free radicals. (See Chapter 4.)

Extra Scientific Information

- Short-term, strict control of blood glucose in diabetics can control and even partly reverse abnormal vision, according to a 1994 French study. (See *Diabetes Care*, October 1994, pp. 1141-7.)
- A severe "keratomalacia" (dry, soft, ulcerated and perforated cornea) occurred in an emaciated, fifty-seven-year-old alcoholic, who also had acute pancreatitis (inflammation of the pancreas). He was able to see only light and darkness. This eye condition is usually associated with a deficiency of vitamin A. (See *Cornea*, March 1993, pp. 171-3.)

Special Food Sources, Strategies, and Facts

See food lists under "Vitamin A." But concentrate on these foods: kale, collard greens, spinach, mustard greens, okra, broccoli, and brussels sprouts.

Therapy Recommendations

Be sure to take your recommended daily "cocktail" of antioxidants. (See Chapter 4.)

Cross-References

See "Vitamin A," "Vitamin C," "Cataracts," Chapter 4.

FAT

Fat presents us with a classic good news-bad news nutrition story: On the one hand, a certain amount is necessary for body metabolism and energy. But on the other, consuming excessive fat through the diet has been linked to most of our deadliest diseases.

Basic Nutritional Therapy

A low dietary intake of fat has been associated with a variety of health benefits, including lowered risk of heart disease and various cancers, including cancer of the colon, prostate, pancreas, ovary, and breast. (See "Cancers.")

A low-fat diet also benefits the eyes. An ongoing study has been conducted by researchers at the University of Wisconsin Medical School with 5,000 people, ages forty-five to eighty-four, who live in Beaver Dam, Wisconsin. The investigation has revealed that a diet rich in saturated fat and cholesterol may increase the risk of age-related macular degeneration (AMD) by 80 percent. Also, the study has shown that eating a low-fat diet significantly decreases the risk of cataracts. The findings were reported at a seminar sponsored by Research to Prevent Blindness, held in October 1995 in Orlando.

High intake of fat tends to be linked to obesity, an independent health risk for heart disease, cancer, and other problems. (See "Obesity.")

Of course, some fat is necessary for a balanced adult diet. Many nutritionists believe that healthy young children need more fat in their diets than adults do, because of the special food requirements of growing bodies.

One study in support of this position, conducted by Dutch scientists and reported in the November 12, 1994, issue of *Lancet*, focused on more than 500 children who were followed for nine years. Those who had been breast-fed for at least three weeks were half as likely as those who took formula to suffer from neurologic abnormalities, such as coordination problems. The researchers speculated that the long-chain fatty acids in breast milk, which are not present in formula, may contribute more to brain development.

However, this point remains in contention. A May 1995 study reported in the *Journal of the American Medical Association* said that children with high cholesterol levels can safely be placed on low-fat diets to reduce their risk of future disease, without any danger of interfering with their growth or health.

Special Food Sources, Strategies, and Facts

Your daily fat intake should be limited so that no more than 20 to 30 percent of your daily calories comes from fats. Furthermore, you should consume no more than 8 to 10 percent of your daily calories in the form of saturated fats. These include foods with visible fat, such as the fatty portion of meats and chicken, and also fatty animal or dairy foods such as butter, cream, or whole milk. Many dessert pastries are high in saturated fats.

Most of your fat consumption should consist of monounsaturated fats (such as the fat in olive, rape seed, and canola oils, and much of the fat in chicken) and the polyunsaturated fats that are in vegetable and fish oils. A number of studies, including those done by Dr. Scott Grundy, Director of the Center for Human Nutrition, University of Texas Health Science Center at Dallas, have established an association between high consumption of monounsaturated fats and a low incidence of heart disease. Olive oil may actually help protect you from clogging of the arteries!

To calculate your daily portion of fats, you should know that 1 gram of fat translates into 9 calories. If you take in 10 grams of fat with a particular food portion, you are consuming 90 calories of fat. (For more details on figuring the proportion of fats, carbohydrates, and protein in your diet, see the "Carbohydrates" entry.)

Therapy Recommendations

See the discussion under "Basic Nutritional Therapy" and "Special Food Sources."

Cross-References

See "Amino Acids," "Cancers," "Carbohydrates," "Cataracts," "Cholesterol," "Eye Complaints," "Heart Disease," "Meat," "Obesity."

FATIGUE

If you are frequently or chronically tired, you may be suffering from a low-grade infection, anemia, heart disease, insomnia, low blood pressure, hypothyroidism, or any one of a number of other health problems including a lack of regular exercise. See your physician for a full checkup.

However, a food or nutritional deficiency is often at the root of fatigue, as the following discussion demonstrates.

Basic Nutritional Therapy

Nutritional causes of fatigue include the following:

- Obesity
- A failure to eat plenty of complex carbohydrates, the body's main source of fuel (See "Carbohydrates" entry.)
- A generally poor diet, which may lead to inadequate amounts of vitamins, minerals, and other nutrients in the body
- Inadequate blood supplies of iron (anemia)
- Inadequate blood supplies of vitamin B_{12}.
- Hypoglycemia

Extra Scientific Information

- Reduction of body stores of carbohydrate and blood glucose (sugar) is related to feelings of fatigue and the inability to maintain a high-quality athletic performance, according to studies done in 1995 at Virginia Tech. Prevention of carbohydrate depletion in sports begins with a "loaded" training diet of about 60 to 70 percent carbohydrates. If possible, carbohydrate beverages should be consumed during the event at the rate of 30 to 70 grams per hour to reduce the depletion of body carbohydrates. (See

International Journal of Sports Nutrition, June 1995, pp. S13-28.)

- With soccer players, carbohydrate depletion may contribute to fatigue and reduced performance during a match, according to a study at the University of Melbourne in Australia. Soccer players in strenuous competition and training should be encouraged to consume a diet that is relatively high in carbohydrates, at least 55 percent of total daily energy (or calorie) intake. Also, the inclusion of carbohydrate-fortified beverages during and after a match is likely to enhance performance and recovery. (See *Journal of Sports Science*, Summer 1994, pp. S13-6.)

- Taking sustained-release niacin (3,000 milligrams per day) to reduce high cholesterol may result in fatigue, along with other health problems, researchers at the Medical College of Virginia reported in 1994. They concluded that the sustained-release form of niacin should be restricted from use, in favor of the immediate-release type of the drug. (See *Journal of the American Medical Association*, March 2, 1994, pp. 672-7.)

- A diet plan for patients with chronic fatigue syndrome should be based on sound nutritional principles, and fad diets should be avoided, scientists at the Harvard School of Public Health reported in 1993. They found no support for diet therapies that include megavitamin or mineral supplements, royal jelly, or other dietary supplements. Also, they found no proof to support elimination, avoidance, or rotation diets. (See *Archives of Family Medicine*, February 1993, pp. 181-6.)

- The influence on endurance capacity of increasing carbohydrates during prolonged exercise was reported in 1993 by scientists from Loughborough

University, Leicestershire, United Kingdom. They found that runners on a carbohydrate-supplemented diet recovered their endurance capacity within a 22.5-hour period, whereas those on a diet consisting of fat and protein did not. (See *International Journal of Sports Nutrition*, June 1993, pp. 150-64.)

• Animals studied at the University of Texas Health Science Center, San Antonio, showed significant physiologic symptoms of fatigue after being fed a diet deficient in vitamin E. (See *Journal of Applied Physiology*, January 1993, pp. 267-71.)

Special Food Sources, Strategies, and Facts

See discussion and food lists under the "Carbohydrates" entry, especially the material on carbohydrate loading.

Therapy Recommendations

Follow the recommendations in the "Carbohydrates" entry and also in Chapter 4 on antioxidants.

Cross-References

See "Anemias," "Vitamin B," "Carbohydrates," "Iron," "Obesity," Chapter 4.

FIBER, INSOLUBLE

There are two main types of fiber: insoluble and soluble. Although their nutritional benefits overlap somewhat, they offer distinct advantages. This entry will focus on the insoluble type, while the next entry deals with soluble fiber.

Basic Nutritional Therapy

An abundance of insoluble fiber in the diet is beneficial in preventing or treating these health problems:

- Colon cancer
- Diverticulitis
- Constipation
- Obesity

Caution: A high-fiber diet may produce gas, stomach cramps, and other intestinal discomforts unless the new foods are added gradually, over a period of several days.

Extra Scientific Information

- In animal studies conducted at the Hirosaki University School of Medicine in Japan, researchers found that wheat bran diets greatly shortened the transit time of food through the colon, with an increase in stool volume and suppression of fat absorption. These factors suggest the effectiveness of wheat bran in inhibiting the formation of intestinal cancers and also the development of diverticula (pouches) on the large intestine. (See *Tohoku Journal of Experimental Medicine*, August 1995, pp. 227-38.)
- There is a decreased risk of cancer of the esophagus among those who have a high intake of raw fruits and vegetables, especially cruciferous vegetables and dietary fiber, according to a 1995 study done at the National Institutes of Health. The report also revealed an increased risk of this type of cancer among those who are obese. (See *Journal of the National Cancer Institute*, June 7, 1995, pp. 847-8.)

Special Food Sources, Strategies, and Facts

Foods high in insoluble fiber include: wheat bran and whole grain cereals (check the labels for number of grams), corn bran, nuts and seeds, and "crunchy" vegetables like broccoli and carrots.

Insoluble fibers are high in cellulose content and, as the term implies, will not dissolve in water. Consequently, they add bulk to the stool and speed up the movement of food through the intestinal tract.

Therapy Recommendations

Eat a total of 20 to 35 grams of all types of fiber each day. Most people should try to divide their intake evenly between insoluble and soluble fiber.

You can consume your daily quota of at least 10 to 18 grams of insoluble fiber by eating one-third cup of bran cereal, and perhaps a serving of broccoli and a piece of whole wheat bread.

For a more specific example of how high-fiber foods can be included in your menu, see the "Constipation" entry.

Cross-References

See "Cancers," "Carbohydrates," "Constipation," "Diverticulitis," "Fiber, Soluble," "Heart Disease."

FIBER, SOLUBLE

Soluble fiber, which gets its name because it is soluble in water, has functions in the body that overlap to some extent with the insoluble type. (See the "Fiber, Insoluble" entry.) But soluble fiber is different in a number of ways.

Basic Nutritional Therapy

Soluble fiber has been linked in some studies on oat bran and oatmeal consumption to lowering the cholesterol in human blood. As a result, soluble fiber is considered an important food in lowering the risk of atherosclerosis and heart disease. (See "Special Food Sources" for suggestions about insoluble fiber foods.)

Yet, for preventing heart disease, a fiber mix that includes both soluble and insoluble fiber is best. In this connection, the February 14, 1996, issue of the *Journal of the American Medical Association* reported the results of a Harvard School of Public Health study on fiber involving nearly 44,000 men, ages forty to seventy-six. In their six-year investigation, the researchers found that those who consumed the most fiber of all types suffered 35 percent fewer heart attacks than those whose fiber intake was lowest.

The diets of the participants focused on cold cereals, apples, bananas, oranges, peas, cooked carrots, and tomato sauce. Some of these foods are high in soluble fiber, but many others are rich in insoluble fiber. In fact, some of the most popular high-soluble fiber foods, such as dried beans and oats, did not play an important role in these men's diets. In other words, the lower heart attack risk was associated with diets that included plenty of insoluble, as well as soluble, fiber.

Those with the highest fiber intake in this study consumed 25 or more grams of fiber per day, within the limit I am recommending in this book.

The study suggests further that shifting to a fat-free but low-fiber diet may not be enough. It is also important to include low-fat items *and* plenty of high-fiber foods.

There are other benefits from soluble fiber. For one thing, it delays the stomach's emptying into the intestines, which helps stabilize the blood sugars. Also, foods high in soluble fiber, like those high in insoluble fiber, tend to be lower in calories. Soluble fibers tend to create a feeling of fullness, which may aid in weight management.

Extra Scientific Information

- In a twelve-week study at New York Medical College of children with high cholesterol, the addition of soluble fiber (psyllium) to a diet low in saturated fat and cholesterol provided added benefits in the treatment of the children with high cholesterol. (See *Journal of the American College of Nutrition*, June 1995, pp. 251-57.) Other studies have shown that psyllium has a cholesterol-lowering effect for adults.

Special Food Sources, Strategies, and Facts

Good sources of soluble fiber include: oats, oat bran, oatmeal, apples, citrus fruits, dried legumes, beans, lentils, barley, peas, potatoes, raw cabbage, strawberries, and Metamucil®.

Therapy Recommendations

Eat at least 20 to 35 grams of fiber per day, with about half coming from soluble and half from insoluble fiber. (See discussions under "Fiber, Insoluble" and "Constipation" for more details.)

Cross-References

See "Atherosclerosis," "Constipation," "Fiber, Insoluble," "Heart Disease."

FOLIC ACID, FOLATE

Folic acid (also called "folate") is linked to the B vitamin group and has recently been identified as an important player in preventing a number of illnesses. These benefits include:

- Preventing birth defects.
- Reducing risk of heart attacks.

- Reducing risk of strokes.
- Reducing risk of colon cancer.

In a nutshell, if the blood levels of the amino acid homocysteine are high, the risk of these diseases is also high. Taking at least 400 micrograms of folic acid per day, along with vitamins B_6 and B_{12} (especially for those taking 1,000 micrograms or more, or people who are over fifty years of age) is currently the best scientific thinking about dosages.

Folic acid is so important that I have devoted Chapters 2 and 3 of this book to an in-depth treatment of the subject. Please refer to that section for a complete discussion, dietary advice, and my specific recommendations.

GARLIC

Garlic has always been valued for its ability to enhance the flavor of foods, if not for its power to ward off vampires! But a growing body of scientific research shows that there is more to this plant than meets the taste buds.

Basic Nutritional Therapy

Various studies have revealed that garlic may provide health benefits such as these:

- Lowering of total cholesterol and "bad" LDL cholesterol, and raising of "good" HDL cholesterol. There is also evidence that garlic may act as an antioxidant, much like vitamins E and C, by neutralizing free radicals that lead to oxidation of LDL cholesterol and the buildup of plaque in the vessels.
- Lowering of blood pressure.
- The ability to strengthen the immune system, counter infections, kill fungi, and operate as an antiseptic against oral bacteria.

- Functioning as an anticancer agent, especially in animal studies.
- An anticoagulant or anticlotting effect in the blood, which can be protective against thrombosis, the blockage of blood flow by clots, as may happen in a stroke.

Extra Scientific Information

- Eating one fresh clove of garlic (about 3 grams) per day for sixteen weeks resulted in a 20 percent reduction of cholesterol in the blood of male volunteers, aged fifty and above, who were studied by scientists of Kuwait University. There was also an 80 percent reduction in thromboxane in the blood. This is a compound related to the development of thrombosis or blood clotting. Researchers concluded that small amounts of fresh garlic, consumed over a long period of time, may be beneficial in the prevention of thrombosis. (See *Prostaglandins, Leukocytes, and Essential Fatty Acids*, September 1995, pp. 211-12.)
- Studies at Charing Cross & Westminster Medical School in London showed that both water and alcoholic extracts of garlic are very potent inhibitors of blood platelet aggregation (clotting).

Note: Inhibition of clotting can help prevent the formation of clots that may plug up blood vessels and trigger heart attacks or strokes. (See *Current Medical Research and Opinion*, 1995, pp. 257-63.)

- Danish researchers studied the effect of garlic on the aging of human cells. They determined that adding garlic extract to a normal cell culture has some youth-preserving, antiaging effects on human cells. The investigators also noted that other health benefits of garlic may include the following: detoxification (countering poisons), antioxidant activity, antifungal activity, antibacterial activity, and suppression of tumors. (See *Journal of Ethnopharmacology*, July 8, 1994, pp. 125-33.)

- The power of garlic to lower blood lipids is being increasingly recognized, according to researchers at the University of Cambridge Department of Anatomy, United Kingdom. In animal studies, they found that the mechanism in garlic that lowers cholesterol and other lipids may be tellurium, which inhibits liver enzymes. (See *Medical Hypotheses*, April 1995, pp. 295-7.)

Special Food Sources, Strategies, and Facts

Several studies, as well as clinical and anecdotal observations, indicate that as an antibacterial or antiviral agent, raw garlic seems to be effective for many people. For cardiovascular and anticancer benefits, either raw or cooked garlic is effective.

How much is too much? Most people suffer no discomfort from eating up to two cloves of garlic per day. The larger amounts apparently required for therapeutic effects (five or more cloves per day) can result in heartburn, flatulence, and related gastrointestinal problems.

Since garlic is an anticoagulant (it reduces blood clotting), people taking aspirin or other anticoagulant drugs should avoid eating large quantities of garlic.

Despite its many benefits, garlic may trigger some serious health problems in a few cases. In some people, it can cause anemia, weight loss, dermatitis, and asthma. It may also increase the fragility of red blood cells.

But these side effects occur only in a minority of garlic users. As the increasing awareness of the medicinal value of garlic prompts more intense research into chemistry and pharmacology, my expectation is that the benefits of garlic will be more solidly established for the great majority.

Therapy Recommendations

The studies on garlic have concentrated on its ability to lower blood lipids in humans. Most of these reports have shown a positive role for garlic, but not all have indicated the same cholesterol-lowering effect. One problem has been that there is no standard against which we can compare the potency of different preparations of garlic.

At this point, however, enough is known for me to make this recommendation: Start including a clove of garlic per day in your food as a possible preventive medicine against heart disease, high blood pressure, and cancer.

Another suggestion: If you feel a cold coming on, or if you have been exposed to a virus or bacterial infection, try taking a clove of raw garlic. If the nutrient works for you, you may have found a great new preventive tool. If you stay under two cloves a day, it's unlikely you will be any the worse for trying this rather unusual remedy.

Cross-References

See "Cancers," "Heart Disease," "Herbs."

GINSENG

The ginseng root has been used for more than 1,000 years in the Far East, particularly in China, for a number of medicinal purposes, including alleged increases in the sex drive (as an aphrodisiac), overall energy, and bodily strength. Ginseng is also taken as a means of controlling stress. Considerable scientific skepticism has surrounded the claimed benefits of this plant food, but recent medical research confirms some special effects.

Basic Nutritional Therapy

Here are some possible benefits of ginseng, which modern medicine has recognized to varying degrees:

- Ginseng may lessen the intensity of hot flushes and other menopausal symptoms.
- It may strengthen the immune system. (See "Extra Scientific Information.")
- The plant may lower the risk of some cancers. (See "Extra Scientific Information.")
- There is some support for the idea that ginseng operates as an "adaptogen," a new word in the herbal literature that replaces "tonic." In this role, ginseng is believed to build resistance to physical, chemical, and biological stress.
- The root may counter the clogging of the arteries that occurs with atherosclerosis.

Warning: Taking ginseng in large doses or over a long period of time can result in a number of negative side effects including: headaches, nervousness, diarrhea, insomnia, painful or lumpy breasts, vaginal bleeding, skin lesions, or high blood pressure.

Extra Scientific Information

- The immune function of the blood's lymphocytes (a type of white blood cell) tends to decline in elderly people; but taking a saponin derivative found in Panax ginseng counters this decline. (See *Mechanisms of Aging*, August 31, 1995, pp. 43-53.)
- The saponin from ginseng stimulated the healing of wounds and the repair of human tissue in a 1995 study at the Chiba University, Japan. (See *British Journal of Pharmacology*, August 1995, pp. 1188-93.)
- Ginseng users in Korea had a decreased risk of cancer over nonusers in a 1995 Korean investigation.

Specifically, those taking ginseng extracts had fewer cancers of the lip, oral cavity, pharynx, esophagus, stomach, colon, liver, larynx, lungs, and ovaries. But there was no reduction in cancers of the female breast, uterine cervix, urinary bladder, or thyroid gland. (See *Cancer Epidemiology Biomarkers Preview*, June 1995, pp. 401-8.)

- A twenty-eight-year-old woman developed a severe headache after ingesting a large quantity of ethanol-extracted ginseng. Angiograms of her brain showed changes in the arteries that were consistent with cerebral arteritis (inflammation of the cerebral arteries). Researchers felt that the circumstances of this case suggested a causal relationship between the intake of ginseng and the woman's head problems. (See *Neurology*, April 1995, pp. 829-30.)
- There is an absence of compelling research to support the claim that ginseng can improve athletic performance or prolong performance in fatigued humans. (See *Sports Medicine*, October 1994, pp. 229-48.)
- Animal studies in Korea indicated that an extract of ginseng inhibited the development of lung tumors. (See *Planta Medica*, December 1993, pp. 521-4.)
- Large numbers of experiments carried out in small animals have shown that ginseng extracts can prolong swimming time, prevent stress-induced ulcers, increase activity of the immune system, and prevent blood clotting. All of these benefits may contribute to a belief in its "tonic" or "adaptogenic" effect.

The problem is that we are almost totally ignorant about the true impact of ginseng on the human body, at least from published chemical studies. Long-term, controlled, double-blind human experiments must be done to determine its beneficial and possibly harmful effects.

Special Food Sources, Strategies, and Facts

Ginseng can be purchased in teas, roots, chewing gum, capsules, extracts, tablets, powders, cigarettes, candies, and drinks. Unfortunately, the quality and quantity of ginseng varies considerably. The best grades of "Korean Red," a specially "cured" root, retail at more than $20 an ounce.

For specific studies on the amount of ginseng in different products, and some recommendations about their use, see *Consumer Reports*, November 1995, p. 699. One analysis showed that 60 percent of fifty-four ginseng products were worthless, and 25 percent of the sampled products contained no ginseng at all!

Therapy Recommendations

An occasional cup of ginseng tea (say once or twice a week) should have no negative effect on your health and might even increase your defenses against cancer, immune diseases, and other conditions listed in "Basic Nutritional Therapy." But do not exceed this dosage, and do observe the precautions given below.

If you suffer excessive hot flushes during menopause, ginseng tea or some other source of the plant may lessen the symptoms. But since the commercial market for such supplements is largely unregulated, you won't know exactly what you are getting in any bottle or package.

If you do decide to try ginseng or any other herb, observe these precautions:

- Take low doses.
- Allow twenty-four hours between supplement doses so that you can evaluate any change that occurs in your body's tolerance for the drug. Also, you might find you're allergic to it.
- If you experience any unusual reaction, inform your

doctor, and keep empty bottles on hand so that he will know exactly what you have taken.

And remember, ginseng remains a medical enigma, with no unequivocal benefit for humans.

Cross-References

See "Herbs," "Hormones."

HEADACHES

Headaches may occur after you eat or drink a certain food, or when you fail to eat or drink one. For more, see "Basic Nutritional Therapy."

Basic Nutritional Therapy

Nutrition-related headaches are a very personal matter. Certain individuals react negatively to certain foods or drinks, while others don't. For this reason, if you tend to experience recurrent headaches, it's important to note when the symptoms occurred and also whether you just ate or drank something. By being observant, you will be more likely to notice a connection between your diet and your pains.

Here are some illustrations of different types of foods, drinks, and herbs that may cause headaches:

- Caffeine. Some people are so sensitive to caffeine that just a little bit will cause a headache or other reaction. Others get headaches from taking in too much. Most people who are regular coffee or tea drinkers experience headaches along with other withdrawal symptoms for at least a day or two when they abruptly try to eliminate caffeine from their diets.
- Food additives, including those containing sulfites.
- Aspartame (in NutraSweet® or Equal®).

Prior to its approval in 1981, aspartame underwent more testing than any other food additive in the history of the FDA. Despite that degree of study, there were more than 3,000 consumer complaints by 1987. Users reported such adverse symptoms as headaches, dizziness, skin rashes, and nausea. Yet after evaluating 517 reports of such aspartame-related symptoms, the Centers for Disease Control came to the conclusion that the symptoms could not be linked to aspartame consumption. (See *Environmental Nutrition*, December 1987.)

- Wine. (See the "Wine" entry.)
- Ginseng. (See the "Ginseng" entry.)

Another source of headaches is hunger. If you tend to get headaches late in the afternoon, and you also are low on glycogen (blood sugar) at those times because you never eat a snack, it's almost certain that your discomforts are linked to your diet. Try a low-calorie, low-fat snack, such as a piece of fruit, to tide you over to the next meal.

Therapy Recommendations

If you regularly suffer from headaches, including migraines, take a close look at your diet. If the pains occur right after you eat or drink a certain food or beverage, try eliminating that item from your diet. Also, ask your physician if there is scientific data linking the food or drink you suspect with headaches.

Cross-References

See "Caffeine," "Ginseng," "Wine."

HEART DISEASE

This topic is dealt with in some detail in other sections of the book. In particular, see the entries "Atherosclerosis,"

"Cholesterol," "Fiber," and the various references under "heart disease" in the index.

HERBS

In non-Western societies, plant extracts, including many herbal remedies, have been used effectively for thousands of years to treat various diseases and medical complaints. While these remedies can never be a substitute for the scientific techniques and drugs we have developed in medicine in the West, they can often be strong supplements to our health programs.

One problem at the present time is that we have little solid, scientific information about many of these herbal cures and remedies. Western research is only beginning to plumb the depths of these treatments. Another problem is that the U.S. Food and Drug Administration (FDA) is not involved in regulating the manufacture and sale of these supplements. As a result, consumers often don't know exactly what they are getting.

Reminder: The FDA requires extensive clinical studies in human beings before granting approval to a drug. It's unlikely this will happen with herbal remedies because drug companies usually won't fund such research.

Even with these limitations, however, some herbs can add a great deal to your personal food program and health plan.

Basic Nutritional Therapy

The following is a summary of herbs that might help you, and also those that might hurt. This list was compiled by physicians at the Cooper Clinic from a number of sources, including studies in medical journals and investigations conducted by *Consumer Reports*.

Herbs That Might Help You

Chamomile:

- Used for indigestion, menstrual cramps, minor infections, and illnesses.
- Derived from the flowering portion of flowers in the daisy family.
- The drug is taken as a strong tea, which must be made fresh from the herb (volatile oil). It should be prepared in a covered vessel and steeped for a long time. Still, the tea will contain only 10 to 15 percent of the volatile oil originally present in the plant.
- Should be avoided by those with allergies to ragweed, daisies, asters, or chrysanthemums. But reports of negative side effects from chamomile are lacking in the scientific literature.

Echinacea:

- Soothes sore throats and aids in wound healing.
- Used as an "immunity booster."
- Derived from the daisy family.
- May help with immune resistance by stimulating white blood cells (phagocytosis).
- Should be avoided by those with allergies to daisies and those suffering from TB, collagen disorders, and multiple sclerosis.

Feverfew:

- Useful in reducing the frequency and severity of migraine headaches. A British study did suggest some effect in treating migraines if taken daily.
- May be of value in treating menstrual irregularity, stomachache, and especially fevers.
- Available in tablet and capsule form, but tablets vary widely in potency.

Garlic:

- Used to lower high cholesterol.
- A 1993 study reported that one-half to one clove daily could lower total cholesterol by 9 percent.
- Active ingredient is allicin.
- Enteric-coated pills help cut odor.
- May have anticoagulant effect. As a result, patients on aspirin, warfarin, or other blood-thinning drugs should avoid it.
- May cause heartburn and flatulence.

(For more details, see the "Garlic" entry.)

Ginger:

- Taken as a tea or in capsule form.
- Used to control nausea, though one recent report indicated that it had no effect on postoperative nausea with surgery patients.
- May help with motion sickness if taken twenty minutes before travel, and repeated every two or three hours as needed.
- No side effects with moderate doses (2 to 4 grams), though very high doses may have an anticoagulant effect and may cause depression of the central nervous system and cardiac irregularities.

Ginkgo biloba:

- Used to improve circulation and treat peripheral vascular disease.
- May enhance blood flow to the brain, according to some studies.
- May improve concentration and memory, particularly in the elderly.
- May enhance blood flow to the legs. As a result, some people use it for cramps.

- Also functions as an antioxidant (free radical scavenger) and helps inhibit lipid peroxidation of cell membranes (a process that leads to atherosclerosis, or clogging of the arteries).

Hawthorn:

- Used for heart disease.
- Substances in the plant may dilate blood vessels, thereby lowering their resistance and increasing blood flow.
- May lower blood pressure.
- May act as smooth muscle relaxer in coronary (heart) vessels.
- *Warning:* This herb should *not* be used as a substitute for conventional therapy.

Final note: Further scientific studies are urgently needed for a drug as potentially valuable as this one.

Milk thistle:

- Used for hepatitis and cirrhosis of the liver.
- Human studies encouraging, not conclusive.
- Silymarin is the ingredient that may confer some protection to the hepatocyte (liver cell) membranes.
- Best administered by injection.

Saw palmetto:

- Used for BPH, or benign prostatic hyperplasia (non-malignant enlargement of the prostate), but not FDA approved.
- Prescribed widely until the 1950s.
- Interferes with testosterone metabolism ("anti-androgenic") and has a slight anti-inflammatory effect.
- May improve urinary flow in men with BPH.

Valerian:

- Used to improve sleep.
- May have a mild sedative and tranquilizing effect, and used as a treatment for restlessness due to nervous conditions.
- Operates through a pathway mediated by the central nervous system.
- Taken as a tea, tincture, or capsule.
- Very unpleasant odor. Some have described it as smelling like a locker room, old socks, cheese.

Warning—Herbs That Might Hurt You

Comfrey:

- Used externally for treating minor skin ailments.
- Variety of forms: tea, tincture, capsule, lotion. *Caution:* Using it internally is definitely hazardous to your health.
- Documented cases of liver problems with increased risk of cirrhosis.
- Consumption during pregnancy may increase risk of liver damage in the fetus.
- Animal studies have shown lung, kidney, and gastrointestinal problems.
- Used in folk medicine in the form of an externally applied poultice for healing wounds.
- Restricted availability in Australia, Canada, Great Britain, and Germany.

Ephedra (Mahuang):

- Used for weight control, energy enhancement.
- Relieves constriction and congestion associated with bronchial asthma.
- Also called "epitonin."
- Contains ephedrine, pseudoephedrine.

- Can increase blood pressure and heart rate, cause palpitations, and lead to strokes.
- Dangerous for people suffering from heart conditions, hypertension, diabetes, or thyroid disease.
- Herbal products containing ephedrine have been banned in Florida and restricted in some other states because of deaths associated with taking ephedrine-containing supplements. Many diet pills, prescription drugs, and over-the-counter medications for allergies, colds, and asthma contain ephedra.

Warning: Stay away from all herbal supplements containing this substance. Use medications containing it only after getting clearance from your physician.

Lobelia:

- In large doses, causes vomiting.
- Used to increase energy and as a stimulant.
- Sometimes called "Indian tobacco." Produces a mild, legal "high" analogous to that caused by smoking marijuana.
- Pharmacologically, this herb is similar to nicotine, though less potent. Supposedly it can produce feelings of mental clarity, happiness, and well-being.
- Large doses can decrease blood pressure, with a resulting increase in heart rate and skin pallor. In some cases, coma and death have resulted.

Warning: Any use of lobelia is definitely not recommended.

Yohimbe:

- Touted as being able to improve male potency.
- Taken from the bark of an African tree.

- Probably ineffective in delivering on traditional claims.
- An overdose can cause hypotension (excessively low blood pressure), increased nerve stimulation, gastrointestinal upsets, paralysis, or even death.
- Sales are prohibited in Georgia.
- This drug should not be taken by people suffering from low blood pressure, diabetes, or diseases of the heart, liver, or kidney.

Extra Scientific Information

- Swedish scientists at Uppsala University examined the power of plants used in traditional Swedish medicine to treat inflammatory disease and wounds. They found that the following plants were effective to one degree or another: *Calluna vulgaris, Corylus avellana, Geum urbanum, Juniperus communis, Polygonum aviculare, Potentilla erecta, Salix caprea, Geum rivale, Solanum dulcamara, Symphytum x uplandicum,* and *Vaccinium vitis-idaea.* (See *Journal of Ethnopharmacology,* October 1995, pp. 61-76.)

Therapy Recommendations

See "Basic Nutritional Therapy" for an overview of the relative safety and effectiveness of various herbs.

I see no problem in experimenting with the safe herbs listed above to see whether they work with specific health problems. But remember: These substances are diluted drugs. As such, they are potentially quite powerful; especially when taken in large doses, they may be dangerous.

To protect yourself, you should alert your physician about your intention to try herbal remedies and get his or her clearance, particularly if you are suffering from a health problem. Some of these herbs can interact with other drugs or medications you are taking.

Also, observe the precautions that have already been listed in the discussion under "Ginseng":

* Take low doses.
* Allow twenty-four hours between supplement doses so that you can evaluate any change in your body's tolerance for the herb.
* If you experience any unusual reactions, inform your doctor immediately, and keep empty bottles on hand to show your doctor exactly what you have taken.

Cross-References

See "Garlic," "Ginseng," "Hormones."

HIGH BLOOD PRESSURE (HYPERTENSION)

Controlling high blood pressure often involves a great deal more than focusing on diet. But your food plan can certainly play a major role as you try to overcome this problem. For a more complete treatment of high blood pressure, see my book *Overcoming Hypertension* (Bantam, 1991).

Basic Nutritional Therapy

Here are some key nutritional guidelines to keep in mind as you work to control your blood pressure:

* Stay at your optimum weight. Even a few extra pounds can elevate your blood pressure. Any extra body fat, especially upper body fat, increases your risk.
* Limit the sodium in your diet. If you have no problem with high blood pressure, you should still stay between 2,400 and 3,000 milligrams per day. But if you do have a problem, take in less than 2,400 milligrams (2.4 grams) per day. (See "Salt" entry.)

Not everyone's blood pressure is salt-sensitive. But significant numbers of adults do experience an increase in blood pressure with an increase of sodium or salt.

Note: Salt is made up of 40 percent sodium and 60 percent chloride. If you know only the number of grams of salt in a particular food, multiply that amount by 40 percent, or 0.40, to get the number of grams of sodium.

- Take in plenty of potassium every day, especially if you are on a blood pressure medication, such as a diuretic. This type of drug will cause you to lose water and body salts. (See the "Electrolytes" entry.)
- Avoid supplements containing creatine or creatinine. One 1989 study in *Hypertension* reported that hypertensive patients with high creatinine levels (creatine is muscle tissue debris that shows up in the urine) are five times as likely to die of stroke or heart attack as those with low levels.
- Avoid caffeine. It can raise blood pressure on a short-term basis.
- Eat a diet low in saturated fats. Various studies recognized by the American Heart Association's Council for High Blood Pressure Research have established a link between elevated blood lipids, such as cholesterol and triglycerides, and high blood pressure.

Note: No more than 20 to 30 percent of your daily intake of calories should come from fats, and most of those calories should come from polyunsaturated and monounsaturated fats. For more on this, see the "Fat" entry.

- Weight your diet heavily in favor of vegetables, which contain plenty of fiber. Vegetarians tend to have lower blood pressure than nonvegetarians. You should also include other high-fiber foods in your daily food program, including wheat bran cereals.

* Take in substantial amounts of calcium every day, at least 1,000 milligrams, and preferably closer to 1,500. (See the "Calcium" entry.)

Scientific studies have shown that oral calcium supplements can lower the pressure of some patients with mild or moderate hypertension.

* Avoid natural licorice that contains glycyrrhizic acid. This food tends to raise blood pressure. (See "Licorice.")
* Get involved in a smoking cessation program.
* Consider taking coenzyme Q10 supplements, which have lowered blood pressure in some instances. (See "Coenzyme Q10.")
* Avoid alcohol, which is associated with higher blood pressure. If you simply can't give it up, at least limit yourself to no more than one average-size mixed drink a day if you are a man, or three mixed drinks a week if you are a woman. (See "Alcohol.")
* Get involved in a regular aerobic exercise program.
* Use relaxation and biofeedback therapy.

Special Food Sources, Strategies, and Facts

See the discussion under "Basic Nutritional Therapy."

Therapy Recommendations

See the discussion under "Basic Nutritional Therapy," and also my book *Overcoming Hypertension.*

Cross-References

See "Alcohol," "Atherosclerosis," "Calcium," "Coenzyme Q10," "Electrolytes," "Fat," "Fiber," "Heart Disease,"

"Herbs," "Licorice," "Salt," "Wine." Also, consult my book *Overcoming Hypertension* (Bantam, 1991).

HORMONES

As she enters the premenopausal years, nearly every woman finds herself asking this question: Should I take hormones when I go through menopause?

Most physicians now recommend hormone replacement therapy (HRT), or as it is sometimes called, estrogen replacement therapy (ERT). There are three reasons for this position:

- To reduce, if not completely eliminate, the menopausal symptoms, particularly hot flushes, or "flashes" as some women call them.
- To reduce the cardiovascular problems associated with the menopausal years. (Probably, these are due to a reduction in the "good" or HDL cholesterol.)
- To prevent or perhaps even reverse osteoporosis, or brittle-bone disease.

Note: For years, it has been known that post-menopausal estrogens, if taken alone, increase substantially the risk of cancer of the uterus. For that reason, progestins (progesterone or Provera) are used in a cyclical fashion in conjunction with estrogen.

Until recently, there was some discussion as to the benefit for the heart of the combined estrogen-progestin (HRT) therapy. An article published in the August 15, 1996, issue of the *New England Journal of Medicine*, followed 59,337 women in the Nurses Health Study of sixteen years. Even though heart problems were rare in these women (only 271 documented heart attacks), both estrogen and the combined estrogen-progestin therapies were helpful.

The risk of heart disease was 61 percent lower in

post-menopausal women taking the combination of hormones, compared with those who took no hormones. Also, the risk was 40 percent lower in those taking estrogen alone.

These findings indicated that combined therapy was just as effective as straight estrogen, but the numbers were not large enough for a definite conclusion that the combination is actually better.

Studies have shown that estrogen replacement can protect post-menopausal women against osteoporosis and decrease the incidence of spine fractures by 70 percent and hip fractures by 50 percent. It is most beneficial when started in the first few years after menopause and may be of some value in treating women with established osteoporosis (see *Medical Letter*, 34:101, 1992). There are also promising new non-hormone drugs available for treating osteoporosis including alendronate (Fosamax-Merck), salmon calcitronin nasal spray (Miacalcin-Sandoz), and slow-release sodium flouride.

Despite these advances, estrogen still remains the treatment of choice in preventing osteoporosis and providing protection against heart disease. But there remains the question about the increased risk of cancer with estrogen. Estrogen combined with progestin brings the risk of uterine cancer down to that of the general population, but either HRT or ERT tends to increase the risk of breast cancer according to the Nurses Health Study.

The study also showed that the increased risk of breast cancer associated with five or more years of post-menopausal hormone therapy was greater among older women. This study suggests that women over fifty-five years of age should consider carefully the higher risks of therapy, especially if they have used hormones for five or more years. (See *New England Journal of Medicine*, 332:1589-93, 1995.)

To sum up this link between hormones and breast cancer: Estrogen alone, estrogen plus progesterone, and progestin alone all appear to raise the risk of breast cancer.

Does the post-menopausal woman have an option, other than hormone or estrogen replacement therapy?

I believe she does. Of the three major problems that occur with menopause (i.e., hot flushes and mood changes, increased risk of heart disease, and increased risk of osteoporosis), the last two often can be controlled with a good exercise program plus adequate calcium intake.

The hot flushes and other vasomotor symptoms cannot be eliminated with exercise, but exercise plus a wise nutrition strategy may provide some answers. In the first place, I'm convinced the hot flushes are less intense and shorter in duration in highly conditioned women. As for nutrition, a wise food strategy may not only help control menopausal symptoms for many women, but may also offer some protection against breast and uterine cancer. Specifically, it may be possible to reduce menopausal symptoms and minimize cancer risks by relying more on "phytoestrogens," or the weak estrogen-like compounds that can be found in many common foods.

Basic Nutritional Therapy

As we have seen, hormone replacement therapy (HRT) protects women against these diseases that can threaten during the onset of menopause or "perimenopause." Also, HRT may be required after menopause, or in other circumstances when the estrogen-progesterone balance is disturbed.

In addition to HRT, a number of plant-derived hormones, including the so-called "phytoestrogens," may have a beneficial impact on the delicate hormonal balance in the female body. In particular, these nutrition-based treatments have been shown to help with symptoms of menopause such as hot flushes, and may also be of value in preventing breast cancer. (See "Food Sources.")

My position on both HRT and the use of food-derived phytoestrogens is summed up in the following strategy, which applies to women with normal reproductive organs.

Caution: Before you take any of the following steps, you should get clearance from your physician. Also, those who have had their ovaries removed, who have been diagnosed as having a hormone imbalance, or who have confirmed osteoporosis must work with their physicians to develop a more personal medical approach.

Step 1. Have your bone density checked by age forty. If the density is lower than 90 percent as predicted for your age, your physician will prescribe treatment, such as increased weight-bearing exercise, higher intake of vitamin D and calcium, or specific bone-building medications. If it is above 90 percent, you should be able to wait for another bone-density test at menopause.

Step 2. Have your bone density checked again at menopause. At this stage of life, estrogen and progesterone levels tend to drop. When this happens, a woman becomes more susceptible to the diseases and conditions already mentioned, including heart disease, osteoporosis, and the uncomfortable symptoms of menopause such as mood changes and hot flushes. If your bone-density level is still above 90 percent at menopause, you may not need HRT to prevent osteoporosis. But you may need hormone replacement therapy for prevention of heart disease, particularly if there is a strong family history of heart disease, or if you have several of the major coronary risk factors.

A thorough physical exam will reveal if your risk of heart disease has increased with the arrival of menopause. For example, when a woman's hormone levels drop, her "bad" or LDL cholesterol may rise and the "good" or HDL cholesterol frequently declines.

Step 3. If your physician determines that you are not at increased risk for osteoporosis or heart disease, but you are experiencing hot flushes and other menopausal symptoms, consider using some nonhormonal medications, or including more plant-derived phytoestrogens (isoflavones) in your diet.

The low levels of these phytoestrogens found in such vegetables as soybeans, wild yams, corn, apples, carrots, barley, and oats will probably increase the sex hormones in your body only slightly because they have relatively "weak" estrogen activity, according to chemical analyses. But the rise in hormones may be just enough to "silence" the receptors in your cells that cause menopausal symptoms.

Wild yams are known to have a substance in them comparable to progestin, the hormone found in progesterone. This was discovered several years ago when researchers noted that some underdeveloped countries seem to have a type of natural birth control. Later, they discovered that the food most likely to produce this effect was wild yams, which contain progestin, a hormone in birth control pills.

Some physicians are now using a topical wild yam cream (usually applied on the insides of the upper thighs) as a means of controlling menopausal symptoms. Many women who still have their uterus and must take a combination of estrogen and progestin (progesterone), have found the side effects from the progestin unacceptable. These include weight gain, irritability, swelling of the extremities, and mood swings. Yet they have found some relief from their menopausal symptoms by discontinuing their HRT and relying strictly upon the wild yam cream.

If you are having problems with your HRT, you might want to discuss this approach with your physician. Wild yam cream is a nonprescription drug, but I would advise against taking it without a physician's recommendation.

A further word of caution: Some health food stores sell

an extract of wild yam that is billed as DHEA (the natural hormone substance that either acts independently or is converted by the body into sex hormones and other steroids). But DHEA exists in plants only in a precursor form, not in its fully formed state. The body itself cannot convert any plant extract into DHEA. Also, in one experiment with rats, fourteen out of sixteen on DHEA developed liver cancer. (See *University of California at Berkeley Wellness Letter*, January 1996.)

So long as you don't overdose on these foods, you should not have to worry about taking in so many phytoestrogens that you upset the basic hormonal balance in your body. (See "Food Sources.")

Caution: Be sure to let your doctor know if you plan to try this nutritional approach. Since food-based hormones are impossible to measure in a normal daily diet, you must be checked periodically to see what is happening in your body. These nutrients can have a decidedly different impact on the systems of different people.

Extra Scientific Information

- Chemicals in certain foods, such as soybean products, certain vegetables, whole grain cereals, seeds, and probably berries and nuts, are converted in the human body into hormone-like compounds. These compounds are capable of antioxidant action and also "weak" estrogen activity (see the above discussion on this topic), reported Finnish researchers from the University of Helsinki in 1995.

The investigators also said that these plant compounds operate in the body in ways that make them strong candidates as natural cancer-protective agents. Furthermore, epidemiologic studies show that the highest levels of these compounds in the diet are found in countries with a low incidence of cancer. (See *Environmental Health Perspectives*, October 1995, Supplement, pp. 103-12.)

- Phytoestrogens (or isoflavones) not only reduce the risk of breast and prostate cancers, they may also lower total serum cholesterol, and at the same time, raise "good" or HDL cholesterol. Also, they may slow bone-density loss in women after menopause and lessen menopausal symptoms like hot flashes and mood swings. But most important, these positive benefits occur without the known carcinogenic (cancer-causing) risk of more concentrated drug therapy, such as HRT. (See *Environmental Nutrition*, April 1995.)
- Dietary phytoestrogens may lessen the adverse effects of obesity on the development of post-menopausal breast cancer, according to a report from the Northern California Cancer Center in 1995. (See *Cancer Causes and Control*, November 1995, pp. 567-73.)
- The beneficial effects of dietary soybean protein (vs. animal protein) on blood lipids, such as the lipoproteins in cholesterol, and on atherosclerosis (the clogging of the arteries that leads to heart attacks) has been known for about fifty years, according to scientists at the Bowman Gray School of Medicine of Wake Forest University.

In an animal study involving rhesus monkeys, researchers found that the phytoestrogens in soy protein reduced "bad" LDL cholesterol by 30 to 40 percent and significantly increased "good" HDL cholesterol. Also, total cholesterol went down by 20 percent in the males and by 50 percent in the females. Furthermore, the phytoestrogens had no adverse effects on the reproductive systems of either the male or female monkeys. (See *Journal of Nutrition*, January 1996, pp. 43-50.)

- Populations consuming soybeans have reduced rates of breast, colon, and prostate cancers, possibly due to the presence of two estrogenic "isoflavones," called "genistein" and "daidzein."

One animal study proved that genistein and daidzein suppress certain chemical reactions in the body induced by a cancer-producing agent. (See *Cancer Letter*, August 16, 1995, pp. 125-33.)

- Australian scientists confirmed in a 1995 report that plants contain compounds called phytoestrogens, which have an estrogen-like action. Their study at the Brighton Medical Clinic focused on fifty-eight post-menopausal women with an average age of fifty-four years, who experienced at least fourteen hot flushes per week. During the study, the women's daily diets were unchanged, were supplemented with soy flour, or were supplemented with wheat flour.

The results: Hot flushes decreased by 40 percent in the soy flour group and by 23 percent in the wheat flour group. Also, the soy flour group experienced a particularly rapid response, which continued for a longer period than the relief experienced by the other groups. (See *Maturitas*, April 1995, pp. 189-95.)

- In a 1995 review article on osteoporosis in Asia, the authors noted that a soy diet, which is consumed in large quantities by Asians, reduces mortality (death) in breast and prostate cancers because it contains weak estrogens.

But the weak phytoestrogens in this diet require further study to show if they also reduce the rate of osteoporosis, the researchers said. (See *Chung Hua I Hsueh Tsa Chih [Taipei]*, March 1995, pp. 209-13.)

- Some 300 plants with estrogen-like activities have been identified. Products made from soybeans (tofu, for instance) have received the most attention because they appear to pack a more potent estrogenic punch.

Phytoestrogens protect against breast cancer by blocking some of the body's naturally occurring estrogen, thus acting as a kind of "anti-estrogen." It's possible for a postmenopausal woman to get an estrogen "lift" without raising her cancer risk by consuming phytoestrogens.

In men, phytoestrogens appear to block testosterone, which can stimulate the growth of prostate cancer. This is accomplished without any "feminizing" effects. (See *Tufts Newsletter*, Vol. 12, no. 12, February 1995.)

- Flaxseed contains high levels of phytoestrogens, according to a study reported by the U.S. Food and Drug Administration in 1995. Also, chaparral, associated with toxic hepatitis, contains substances similar to estrogenic compounds, but the FDA considers chaparral unsafe for human consumption. My recommendation: Stay away from chaparral! Despite the potential dangers, chaparral products have been marketed as dietary supplements. (See *Proceedings of the Society for Experimental Biology and Medicine*, January 1995, pp. 6-12.)
- Flax products contain high levels of "lignan" phytoestrogens, which are structurally similar to human estrogen. Many lignans have been reported to have antitumor, antioxidant, and weak estrogenic powers. Flaxseed products are currently being marketed as dietary supplements and as food constituents. While no adverse effects have been documented so far, the

long-term effect of high consumption of this product is unknown. (See *P.S.E.B.M.*, Vol. 208, 1995.)

- Ginseng has been recommended for its estrogenic or female-hormone effects. But an analysis published in "The Honest Herbalist" (*Peismal Communication*, January 29, 1991) concluded that there is no experimental evidence to support such activity.

- Dong quai, the root of a Chinese plant, has been recommended by modern herbalists for the treatment of a multitude of female problems, including menstrual cramps, irregular or retarded flow, and relief of menopausal symptoms. Yet large doses cause undesirable side effects, and currently, there is not sufficient clinical evidence to support its effectiveness. So I can't recommend its use. (See "The Honest Herbalist.")

- Black cohosh comes from a North American forest plant commonly called snakeroot or rattleweed. A claimed estrogenic effect to stimulate menstruation could not be verified in comprehensive experiments on mice in 1960. (*Arzneimittel-Forschung* 10:514-20, 1960.) Subsequent studies in rats have shown some estrogenic activity, but there are no studies yet on humans. Still, black cohosh is being used in Europe to treat premenstrual syndrome symptoms (PMS), painful menstruation, and menopausal symptoms. Though further studies on this potentially useful drug are warranted, I can't recommend it at this point. (See "The Honest Herbalist.")

- Blue cohosh, also known as papoose root or squawroot, is a perennial herb. It has been used since at least 1813 as an "Indian herb medicine" for a multitude of medical problems, including uterine stimulation and inducing menstruation.

Warning: Because of its potential toxic effects, including constriction of the coronary blood vessels, blue cohosh cannot be dismissed as either inactive or harmless. It should not be used for medical self-treatment.

Special Food Sources, Strategies, and Facts

See "Therapy Recommendations" and "Basic Nutritional Therapy."

Therapy Recommendations

Foods and herbs that are known to contain phytoestrogens and estrogen-like substances—and which you may include as part of a well-balanced diet—include: soybean products, wild yams, corn, apples, carrots, barley, oats, whole grain cereals, nuts, and berries. Flaxseed and possibly black cohosh can be used with close medical supervision. Ginseng, dong quai, unicorn roots, blue cohosh, and chaparral cannot be recommended. See the "Ginseng" entry for my position on this root. Special supplements or large doses for the products mentioned above vary among individuals and must be professionally prescribed. But there is at least one exception: Two ounces of soy protein, taken daily in the form of one-half cup of tofu, one-third cup of soy flour, or one cup of soy milk, have been associated with positive health changes, without the side effects of drug therapy.

Cross-References

See "Atherosclerosis," "Calcium," "Ginseng," "Heart Disease," "Herbs," "Osteoporosis."

IMMUNITY

This entry will provide a brief summary of immunity, with some of the latest scientific findings. The subject of immunity has been treated in some detail in Chapter 3 of this book, and also in my *Antioxidant Revolution*. For further discussions, refer to the other sources mentioned in "Cross-References" below.

Basic Nutritional Therapy

There are many nonnutritional ways to keep your immune system in good working order, such as getting regular exercise and sleep. But what you eat can also impact your ability to ward off infection and disease.

Your first nutritional line of defense should be a complete "antioxidant cocktail," such as I recommended in Chapter 4.

For example, the "bad" or LDL cholesterol would not be "bad" if it were not oxidized by free radicals (unstable oxygen molecules). Ordinarily, LDL cholesterol is used in many normal body functions and is essential for life. Yet the combination of excess LDL cholesterol and excess free radicals results in a destructive interaction (an "oxidizing" action). The resulting oxidized cholesterol is then deposited in the lining of the vessels, and a buildup of plaque causes arteriosclerosis and heart disease.

The antioxidant vitamins C and E are especially important in this scenario. They attack and neutralize the excess free radicals and allow those that remain to go about their normal function of fighting bacteria and bolstering your immune system. Also, this action will keep your white blood cells (particularly immunity-bolstering macrophages) from being wasted in trying to counter the presence of oxidized LDL cholesterol. (See Chapter 4.)

In addition to taking antioxidants, you can strengthen your immune system by eating a well-balanced diet high in vegetables, fruits, carbohydrates, and fiber. (See "Carbohydrates," "Fiber.") Also, there are scientific reports indicating that immunity can be bolstered in certain situations by eating a restricted protein diet, taking in polyunsaturated fatty acids (especially fish oil), and reducing obesity. (See "Extra Scientific Information.")

Extra Scientific Information

- Dietary supplementation with polyunsaturated fatty acids may prevent suppression of the immune system, and thereby improve the body's ability to repair itself after trauma injury. (See *Nutrition*, January-February 1995, pp. 1-11.)
- Excess weight is associated with impairments in the human immune defense mechanisms. (See *Nutrition Review*, February 1994, pp. 37-50.)
- In animal studies conducted at Michigan State University in 1993, fish oil was fed to mice for three weeks before they were made to hemorrhage. The fish oil helped maintain normal "macrophage" (white blood cell) functions and thus enhanced immunity following the hemorrhage. (See *Archives of Surgery*, January 1993, pp. 15-21.)
- Researchers at the University of Munich, Germany, noted in a 1995 report that a continuing high blood cholesterol after a heart transplant can result in an ongoing oxidation of LDL. The oxidized LDL then is "eaten" by white blood cells that sense a destructive foreign presence in the body. Finally, the LDL-white blood cell combination lodges in the artery wall of the new heart grafts to form the plaque of atherosclerosis.

In the study, only 12 percent of patients who were given a medication to lower total and "bad" LDL cholesterol experienced vessel disease, in contrast to 24 percent who did not receive the medication. (See *Kidney International Supplement*, December 1995, pp. S52-5.)

- Dietary protein restriction improved the condition of patients with failure of kidney transplants by suppressing the immune-related renin-angiotensin system. (See *Kidney International Supplement,* December 1995, pp. S102-6.)

Special Food Sources, Strategies, and Facts

See "Cross-References."

Therapy Recommendations

See "Basic Nutritional Therapy" and also Chapter 4.

Cross-References

See "Vitamin C," "Carbohydrates," "Vitamin E," "Fat," "Fiber," "Protein," Chapter 4.

INSOMNIA

About 65 million adult Americans, or 36 percent of the population, complain of poor sleep. Of these, one-fourth have insomnia on an ongoing basis.

These chronic insomniacs report problems with concentration, memory, and the ability to cope with minor irritations. They also have two and one-half times more fatigue-related auto accidents than good sleepers. (See *Drug Safety,* October 1995, pp. 257-70.)

Various techniques and treatments have worked to some degree to produce good sleep. These include relaxation exercises, regular physical exercise (performed at least two to three hours prior to sleep), and in the last resort, physician-supervised sleeping medications.

But for some people, the best treatment for sleeplessness, and certainly the one with the slightest chance of negative side effects, is nutritional therapy.

Basic Nutritional Therapy

Several nutritional approaches may produce satisfying sleep. For example, there are reports that taking magnesium, pyridoxine (vitamin B_6), or thiamin (vitamin B_1) supplements can help insomnia. (See *Australian Family Physician*, letter, March 1994, p. 498.)

Also, many people swear by the essential amino acid tryptophan. Still others vow that a cup of milk, which contains tryptophan, before bed every night is a surefire sleeping potion. (See "Cross-References" below.)

Finally, a number of research projects report success in using melatonin to overcome insomnia. (See the "Melatonin" entry.) But I am not prepared to recommend melatonin until more extensive, long-term studies are completed.

Extra Scientific Information

- A child with a pineal gland tumor (in the brain) experienced severe insomnia, according to Israeli researchers at the Rambam Medical Center in Haifa. An examination showed that the patient had marked suppression of melatonin secretions, and so 3 milligrams of melatonin were given in the evening for two weeks. The result: The child's sleep continuity was restored. (See *Neurology*, January 1996, pp. 261-63.)
- For melatonin-deficient elderly insomniacs, melatonin replacement therapy may be beneficial, according to research done at the Technion-Israel Institution of Technology in Haifa. (See *Sleep*, September 1995.)

Special Food Sources, Strategies, and Facts

See listings under "Amino Acids," "Vitamin B_1," "Vitamin B_6," "Magnesium," "Melatonin."

Therapy Recommendations

There's nothing wrong with drinking a glass of skim milk or consuming foods containing tryptophan just before bedtime. Combine the milk with a carbohydrate such as cereal, and there may be an increase in your blood serotonin level, which can produce calmness, mood stability, reduced stress, and sleepiness.

Moderate doses of magnesium may be of value as well as vitamin B_1 or vitamin B_6.

But before you try melatonin, check with your physician. Also, see my comments under "Basic Nutritional Therapy."

Cross-References

See "Amino Acids, "Vitamin B_1," "Vitamin B_6," "Calcium," "Magnesium," "Melatonin."

IODINE

Most well-balanced Western diets supply plenty of iodine, which is converted into iodide in the gastrointestinal tract. Supplemental iodine is needed only when there is a deficiency of iodine, with accompanying physical problems such as enlargement of the thyroid gland (simple goiter).

This problem afflicts an estimated 200 million people worldwide, mostly in Africa, and all but 4 percent of these cases result from an iodide deficiency. The goiters in this 4 percent, which represents 8 million people, result from overconsumption of plants of the cabbage family and other dietary sources. These foods contain "goitrogen," an antithyroid substance. Surprisingly, excessive intake of iodine also can cause enlargement of the thyroid gland.

Basic Nutritional Therapy

If you include one or two servings of seafood in your diet every week, and in general eat a well-balanced diet with regular servings of dairy products, meat, and poultry, you should easily meet the RDA of 150 micrograms of iodine per day. One gram of iodized salt contains half of your daily iodine requirement.

But if your intake of iodine is inadequate, you may not only develop a goiter, but also a thyroid deficiency called "hypothyroidism." Clinical features of this condition include physical and mental slowness, drowsiness, fatigue, dry skin and hair, intolerance to cold, constipation, and weight gain. In severe cases (myxedema), there is also a puffiness of the face and eyes.

If these symptoms occur with or without enlargement of the thyroid gland, the treatment is supplemental thyroid as prescribed by a physician. A deficiency of iodine or iodide may cause a goiter, but that problem is not corrected with iodine supplementation. In some cases, patients with normal thyroid function and a long-standing goiter develop an overactive thyroid (hyperthyroidism) when given iodine therapy.

A goiter may be reduced in size through thyroid supplementation. If that is not effective, surgical removal may be required.

Extra Scientific Information

- In a 1994 study by the Ministry of Agriculture, Fisheries and Food, London, researchers found that kelp-based dietary supplements contained iodine at levels that would provide a median intake of 1,000 micrograms, if the manufacturers' recommended maximum daily dose of the supplement was taken. This level was far above the United Kingdom's "reference nutrient intake" of 140 micrograms per day for adults, but did not exceed the maximum tolerable intake level of 1,000 micrograms per day established by the Joint Expert Committee on Food Additives. (See *British Journal of Nutrition*, September 1994, pp. 435-46.)

- Dietary iodine deficiency was the primary cause of the endemic goiter problems suffered by children ages six to eighteen in Namibia, according to South African scientists. (See *Central African Journal of Medicine*, March 1994, pp. 60-6.)
- Japanese researchers studied thyroid disease in relation to iodine intake in five coastal areas that produced iodine-rich seaweed. They found that a simple goiter affected nearly 10 percent of the population who consumed an extremely high amount in their diet in the form of seaweed. Such goiters can be corrected by elimination of the seaweed, and normal thyroid function achieved with potassium iodide. (See *Journal of Clinical Endocrinology and Metabolism*, February 1994, pp. 393-7.)

Special Food Sources, Strategies, and Facts

Rich food sources of iodine include: seaweed (kelp), shellfish, and iodized salt.

Therapy Recommendations

Do not take iodine or thyroid supplements unless you are directed to do so by your physician. Radioactive iodine treatments may be prescribed for thyroid problems (hyperthyroidism).

Cross-References

See "Constipation," "Salt."

IRON

Iron has been described as a nutritional double-edged sword. When consumed in moderate quantities and combined with protein-rich foods such as meats, iron plays an essential element in cell metabolism and growth.

But when it is "unleashed" from protein and begins to roam about freely in relatively large quantities through the circulatory system, iron may increase the risk of heart disease and cancer. (See *Stem Cells*, May 1994, pp. 289-303.)

Too little iron in the body, a condition that can occur in a menstruating woman, may result in problems with fatigue and anemia. On the other hand, too much iron may release destructive free radicals, trigger oxidizing actions in the body, and lead to some of the above-mentioned diseases. An iron deficiency may also impair the immune system and make a person more susceptible to disease. In addition, taking iron tablets can cause stomach aches and other symptoms.

One out of every 250 Americans has a genetic condition called "hemochromatosis." These people absorb twice as much iron from their food and supplements as other people do. This extra iron is stored in the liver, brain, pancreas, and heart. But damage does not begin to occur until after age fifty.

At first, there are no symptoms. But later, patients may complain of fatigue, abdominal pain, achy joints, impotence, or symptoms of diabetes (excess thirst and urination). If caught soon enough, damage can be prevented.

Treatment may involve donating blood regularly to get rid of excess iron, and to limit the intake of foods high in iron. Also, iron supplements should be avoided.

Basic Nutritional Therapy

The RDA for adult men, as well as for women who have passed through menopause, is 10 milligrams per day.

The RDA for women who still menstruate is higher: 15 milligrams per day. Also, pregnant and breast-feeding women and growing children typically need more iron. These groups should follow their physicians' instructions about iron intake.

Other groups at particular risk for an iron deficiency include the elderly and certain children. Poor nutrition among older people can result in inadequate stores of iron and lead to lowered immunity, fatigue, and other problems.

As for children, a 1994 study of 196 Spanish students may be instructive. Researchers at the Centro de Salud Velez-Malaga found the following:

- Adolescent girls between thirteen and fifteen were at the greatest risk for iron deficiency.
- Another very high-risk group was six- to seven-year-old boys, followed by thirteen- to fifteen-year-old boys.
- Still another group facing iron deficiency risk was girls ten to twelve years old. (See *Nahrung*, 1994, pp. 192-8.)

A Danish study revealed that young men in their twenties had a satisfactory iron status, but young women of the same age had a higher frequency of iron deficiency. (See *Annals of Hematology*, April 1995, pp. 215-21.)

Extra Scientific Information

- The bioavailability of dietary iron (the ability of the body to obtain it in usable form from food) is a key factor in iron nutrition, according to a Swedish study published in 1995. A diet with much lean meat, ascorbic acid (vitamin C), and a low phytate content (a special kind of fiber) can meet iron requirements in most nonpregnant women. Dietary iron overload will not develop in normal subjects, even with diets having high iron content or high bioavailability. (See *European Journal of Clinical Nutrition*, November 1995, pp. 794-808.)

- A combination of excessive citric acid and ascorbic acid—a synergistic pair of strong iron absorption agents—can be instrumental in causing a damaging increase in iron in aging populations. This iron overload may contribute to heart disease, cancer, diabetes, osteoporosis, arthritis, and other disorders. (See *Biochemical and Molecular Medicine*, February 1995, pp. 1-11.)
- Infants who were exclusively breast-fed for at least seven months had a good iron status at one and two years of age. (See *Journal of Pediatrics*, September 1995, pp. 429-31.)
- High intake of calcium can inhibit absorption of iron by the body if both minerals are present in the same meal, a Canadian study reported in 1995. For this reason, calcium taken as a supplement should always be ingested in a fasting state. (See *Nutritional Review*, March 1995, pp. 77-80.)
- Vitamin C, taken in doses of 2 grams per day for two months, did not have a negative effect on copper or iron metabolisms in humans, according to a 1994 study at the University of Ankara in Turkey. (See *Journal of Nutritional Science and Vitaminology*, October 1994, pp. 401-10.)
- A vegetarian diet rich in soybean products but restricted in animal foods is too limited in iron that can be used by the body, and thus is not adequate to maintain a healthy iron balance in men and women. (See *Journal of Nutrition*, February 1995, pp. 212-19.)
- In a French study, when calcium and phosphorus intake were increased, iron deficiencies often occurred in infants, young children, menstruating

women, and elderly men. (See *Annals of Nutrition Metabolism*, 1994, pp. 192-202.)

- In a 1995 investigation by Swedish scientists at the University of Goteborg, the researchers found that about 30 to 50 percent more iron was absorbed when no milk or cheese was served with lunch or dinner. This result led the investigators to suggest that a separation of time between taking calcium and iron (such as consuming calcium at breakfast and iron at the evening meal) would improve iron nutrition. But again, taking supplemental calcium in a fasting state (i.e., before meals) is best. (See *American Journal of Clinical Nutrition*, January 1995, pp. 97-104.)

- Avoidance of red meat increases the risk of having deficiencies of iron and zinc, according to a 1994 study at the University of Texas Medical Branch, Galveston. (See *Journal of Laboratory and Clinical Medicine*, December 1994, pp. 852-61.)

- The increased iron content in some Chinese foods is due to cooking in metal woks which are 98 percent iron. (See *Journal of the American Dietetic Association*, October 1994, pp. 1153-6.)

- An appropriately planned, well-balanced vegetarian diet can be compatible with an adequate iron status. But restrictive vegetarian diets, such as macrobiotic diets, are associated with iron-deficiency anemia. (See *American Journal of Clinical Nutrition*, May 1994, 5 Supplement, pp. 1233S-7S.)

- In 1992, some Finnish investigators reported that in 2,000 middle-aged men, those with high blood levels of ferritin were more than twice as likely to suffer heart attacks as those with low levels. (See *Circulation*, 86:803, 1992.)

But since then, three of four additional studies that measured ferritin failed to find any link to an increased risk of heart disease. In fact, one study suggested exactly the opposite: The researchers indicated that iron overload is not a risk factor for heart disease and may even be protective against it. (See *Environmental Nutrition*, October 1994.)

Special Food Sources, Strategies, and Facts

Good food sources for iron include: liver, soybeans, peas, whole grain bread, certain enriched cereals (Post 40 Percent Bran® flakes contains 7.5 milligrams per cup, one cup of Total® wheat flakes has 21 milligrams, and toasted wheat germ has more than 10 milligrams per cup), oysters, clams, spinach, and beans. Also, various steak cuts contain fairly high amounts of iron.

Therapy Recommendations

Get your iron from your diet unless you are a pregnant, lactating, or menstruating woman, or you have been diagnosed with an iron deficiency. In such case, you should check with your physician for directions about iron supplements. Feelings of fatigue could be a tip-off to an anemia-related or iron deficiency.

Cross-References

See "Fatigue," "Heart Disease," "Macrobiotic Diet," "Meat," "Zinc," Chapter 4.

VITAMIN K

Vitamin K is a nutrient found in the small intestine where it combines with protein to produce clotting of the blood.

Certain cases of vitamin K deficiency have resulted in a failure of the clotting process and in hemorrhages. In particular, there is a danger that hemorrhages may occur in the brains of newborns who lack sufficient vitamin K.

This vitamin is so prevalent in our food that anyone with a complete diet will usually take in more than enough to produce adequate clotting.

Basic Nutritional Therapy

The maximum RDA for adult men is 80 micrograms of vitamin K per day and for adult women, 65 micrograms. You will get more than enough in one ample serving of green, leafy vegetables, such as the cruciferous vegetables, broccoli or cabbage. One-half cup of broccoli provides 100 micrograms of vitamin K.

Extra Scientific Information

- Blood serum levels of vitamin K are reduced in older individuals and patients with fractures related to osteoporosis. But scientists are not sure whether a lack of vitamin K has any role in causing osteoporosis. (See *Journal of Nutrition*, July 1995, pp. 1812-21.)
- A daily supplementation of 25 micrograms of vitamin K1 was recommended by Dutch scientists in 1993 for breast-fed infants to prevent vitamin K deficiency beyond the neonatal period. This strategy was to prevent the children from hemorrhaging. (See *Journal of Pediatric Gastroenterology and Nutrition*, April 1993, p. 301.)
- To maintain blood serum levels of vitamin K1 within the proper physiological range, repeated administration of low doses is needed beyond one week of age in breast-fed newborns. (See *European Journal of Pediatrics*, January 1993, pp. 72-4.)

Special Food Sources, Strategies, and Facts

Food sources of vitamin K include green leafy vegetables, which are clearly the best dietary sources (50 to 800 mcg per 100 gm of food). Small but significant amounts are present in milk and dairy products, meats, eggs, cereals, and fruits (1 to 50 mcg per 100 gm of food). Also, beef liver is high in this vitamin.

Therapy Recommendations

Just eat the recommended five to seven servings per day of vegetables and fruits and you won't have to worry about vitamin K. (See "Cross-References.")

Cross-References

See "Carbohydrates," "Cruciferous Vegetables," "Fiber."

KETOGENIC DIET

A ketogenic diet consists mostly of fats, with relatively small amounts of carbohydrates and protein. Since the 1920s, it has been used to overcome epileptic seizures in children who do not respond to traditional medications. In addition, the diet has proven to have some effect in treating cancer.

Basic Nutritional Therapy

The theory underlying this diet is that the peculiar weighting of foods toward a very high proportion of fat causes the body to use its own protein for fuel in a metabolic change known as "ketosis." This term refers to the diet's production of ketone chemicals and uric acid in the body.

The most common users of the diet are children between the ages of one and five who do not respond to antiseizure drugs. The children are fed meals with about 80 percent of calories coming from fats and about 20 percent from protein.

Sweets and sugars are not permitted, because adding

even a slight amount of additional carbohydrate may destroy the effect of the diet.

Typically, children stay on the diet for one to three years and then are gradually weaned from it by eating increasing amounts of carbohydrates.

Extra Scientific Information

- A study at the University of Pittsburgh School of Medicine revealed that overweight women on a ketogenic diet performed poorly on a neuropsychological test that required higher order mental processing and flexibility. (See *International Journal of Obesity Related Metabolism Disorders*, November 1995, pp. 811-6.)

- A ketogenic diet may help halt epileptic seizures in selected children who do not respond to medications, according to a study at Johns Hopkins University. The benefits of the diet, especially for those patients who can get no relief from anticonvulsants, include improved control over seizures and reduced behavioral and cognitive side effects from medications. (See *Emilepsia*, 33:1132, 1992.)

- A five-year-old girl who was displaying symptoms of a suspected epileptic syndrome experienced some improvement when her antiepileptic drugs were combined with a ketogenic diet. (See *Epilepsia*, October 1995, pp. 1050-7.)

- When two patients with tumors were placed on ketogenic diets, within seven days their blood glucose (sugar) levels declined to normal, according to researchers at the Case Western Reserve University School of Medicine. Also, a nearly 22 percent average decrease in glucose occurred at the tumor site in both subjects. (A lack of glucose tends to impair the tumor growth.)

One of the patients displayed significant clinical improvements in mood and developed new skills during the study. She stayed on the ketogenic diet for another twelve months and during that period, she remained free of disease progression. (See *Journal of the American College of Nutrition*, April 1995, pp. 202-8.)

- Traditionally, a ketogenic diet is given to drug-resistant children with epilepsy to improve their seizure control. But various studies show that the diet also has the potential to decrease tumor growth, while maintaining the patient's nutritional status.

Preliminary use of the diet suggests a potential in pediatric patients with cancer, according to scientists at the Nutritional Department of Case Western Reserve University. (See *Journal of the American Dietetic Association*, June 1995, pp. 693-7.)

Special Food Sources, Strategies, and Facts
See discussion under "Basic Nutritional Therapy."

Therapy Recommendations
Ketogenic diets should be followed only under the strict supervision of a physician. These food programs are extremely specialized and can have significant, negative impact on your health, or the health of your child, if the mix of fats, carbohydrates, and protein is not precisely observed.

Cross-References
See "Carbohydrates," "Fat."

LICORICE

Licorice is a popular sweet, but it has an established ability to raise blood pressure to dangerous levels.

Symptoms resulting from excessive consumption include headaches, lethargy, sodium and water retention, excessive excretion of potassium, and even heart failure and cardiac arrest. (See *Medical Letter on Drugs and Therapeutics*, 21(7), 1979.)

Basic Nutritional Therapy

Because even relatively small amounts (50 grams or less) of licorice can raise blood pressure, I would recommend that as a general rule, you avoid eating it.

Extra Scientific Information

- Ingestion of licorice may result in retention of sodium and water, hypertension, hypokalemia (low blood potassium levels), alkalosis (too much bicarbonate in the blood), and suppression of the renin-aldosterone system in the kidneys. This is because its main component, glycyrrhizin, is similar in structure to the hormone aldosterone, which regulates the body's water and sodium balance. (See *Netherlands Journal of Medicine*, November 1995, pp. 230-4.)

The authors of this study described the case of a forty-year-old woman who developed severe hypertension and low potassium as a result of prolonged licorice consumption.

- Researchers at the University of Iceland tested whether regular moderate licorice consumption of 50 to 100 grams daily would raise blood pressure. They found that these moderate amounts did indeed raise systolic blood pressure, and they concluded that licorice-induced hypertension may be more common than has been thought. (See *Journal of Human Hypertension*, May 1995, pp. 345-8.)

Special Food Sources, Strategies, and Facts

See "Basic Nutritional Therapy" and "Extra Scientific Information."

Therapy Recommendations

Officially, the extract of licorice root is used only as a flavoring or sweetener. (Its main chemical component, glycyrrhizin, is fifty times sweeter than table sugar!) These are the only two FDA-approved uses of this product.

But licorice has also been used as part of Chinese folklore for 5,000 years as a potent expectorant to relieve the congestion of colds and the flu. It has an anti-inflammatory action that soothes sore throats and ulcers, and may even have anticavity capabilities.

Scientific literature contains significant indication that licorice, even in moderate amounts, can raise blood pressure. As a result, I would recommend that everyone stay away from it.

Cross-References

See "High Blood Pressure."

LONGEVITY

Achieving a longer life span is an ongoing, elusive brass ring pursued by many scientists and nutritionists. But some progress is being made in moving toward this goal, primarily in the area of healthier lifestyles, improved nutrition, and investigations into "subnutrition." Subnutrition involves cutting back significantly on the intake of calories in the hope of increasing personal longevity.

Basic Nutritional Therapy

The three main factors that negatively affect aging are smoking, sedentary living, and obesity. (See *It's Better to Believe*, Thomas Nelson, 1995.)

If you avoid smoking and sidestream smoke, you'll greatly increase your chances to live longer and look younger. If you pursue an active life, with regular endurance exercise and strength training, you will most likely live longer and function physically and mentally at your highest potential until your death. And, if you maintain your ideal weight (a major nutritional ingredient in longevity), you will not only look younger, but you will also eliminate one of the major risk factors for disease.

Another potentially important nutritional factor for longevity is to be sure that you take in regular, relatively high amounts of antioxidants. Preferably, these should come through your diet; but if you can't get enough that way, you should then take supplements. The major antioxidants include vitamin E, vitamin C, and beta-carotene. Also, it's essential for everyone interested in good health and a long life to take regular doses of folic acid. For more on these topics, see Chapters 2 through 4.

Finally, there is growing evidence that cutting back on your calories significantly, by as much as 30 percent of normal daily intake, may increase your life span. (See "Extra Scientific Information" and also my discussion on subnutrition in *It's Better to Believe*, pp. 215ff.)

Extra Scientific Information

- Restriction of calorie intake increases longevity, slows the rate of functional decline, and reduces the incidence of age-related disease in a variety of species, physicians at the University of Texas Health Science Center, San Antonio, reported in 1995. The biological mechanism through which eating less may increase longevity remains unknown, but scientific data suggest that cutting calories alters the functions of cells favorably so that destructive by-products of cellular metabolism are reduced. (See

Clinical Geriatric Medicine, November 1995, pp. 553-65.)

• The decrease of ovary function, which is the cause of menopause, typically accelerates in the decade before menopause; but long-term restriction of calorie intake retards this process. In both animal and human studies, researchers at the University of Texas Health Science Center, San Antonio, are attempting to identify the reasons for changes in brain secretions that may coordinate the life-prolonging response of animals to food restriction. (See *Neurobiology of Aging*, September-October 1995, pp. 837-43.)

Special Food Sources, Strategies, and Facts

See "Cross-References."

Therapy Recommendations

My nutritional suggestions for increasing your chances to live longer can be summed up this way:

• Maintain your ideal weight
• Eat a balanced diet (See discussions under "Amino Acids," "Carbohydrates," "Fat," "Folic Acid," and "Protein.")
• Take in the recommended daily "antioxidant cocktail." See specific recommendations in Chapters 1 through 3
• Try taking in fewer calories than you think you need

Caution: You should not allow your weight to drop too low. If you are a woman, your body fat should not go below 12 percent; if you are a man, your body fat should not go below 7 percent.

Also, a reduction in calories should not make you feel tired or lacking in energy. If you feel run down, fuzzy-headed, or irritable after a week on a low-calorie diet, you are probably taking in too few calories.

Most people should not take in fewer than 1,200 to 1,500 calories per day on a regular basis, unless they are on a diet supervised by a qualified physician or registered dietitian.

Cross-References

See "Vitamin A," "Vitamin C," "Carbohydrates," "Cruciferous Vegetables," "Vitamin E," "Folic Acid," Chapters 1 through 4 of this book, and chapter 13 of my book *It's Better to Believe* (Thomas Nelson, 1995).

MACROBIOTIC DIET

Macrobiotic means "long-lived," but unfortunately the macrobiotic diets followed by many people do not live up to the name.

This radical vegetarian diet has been linked to retarded growth in children and vitamin and mineral deficiencies in adults. Typically, the diet not only eliminates animal foods but also attempts to eliminate as many fats as possible. The most extreme types also downplay dairy products.

This diet is not recommended.

Extra Scientific Information

- Researchers at the Academic Hospital of the Free University of Brussels, Belgium, reported a case of nutritional rickets in a young child who had been on a macrobiotic diet. Rickets results from a lack of vitamin D. (See *Journal of Belgian Radiology*, October 1995, pp. 276-7.)
- Norwegian scientists found cobalamin (vitamin B_{12}) deficiencies in infants who had been on a macrobiotic

diet. (See *Pediatric Research*, August 1994, pp. 194-201.)

- Dutch researchers studied growth patterns in children, from infancy to ten years of age, who were on macrobiotic diets. They found that growth retardation, including inferior height and muscle development, were caused by nutritional deficiencies alone.

As a result of their findings, they modified the children's diets by adding fats, fish, and more dairy products. After these changes, the children experienced a return to more normal growth. (See *European Journal of Clinical Nutrition*, February 1994, Supplement 1, pp. S103-12.)

- Scientists at Wageningen Agricultural University, the Netherlands, studied children on a macrobiotic diet based mainly on whole grain cereals, legumes such as peas and lentils, and vegetables.

The children suffered from a variety of deficiencies of energy, protein, vitamin B_{12}, vitamin D, calcium, and riboflavin. As a result, they experienced retarded growth, wasting of muscle tissue, and slow psychomotor development.

The adults in these families were also subject to nutritional deficiencies. The breast milk from the macrobiotic mothers of these children contained very low levels of vitamin B_{12}, calcium, and magnesium.

The researchers recommended supplementing the macrobiotic diets with fat (a minimum of 20 to 25 grams per day), fatty fish (a minimum of 100 to 150 grams per week), and dairy products (a minimum of 150 to 250 grams per day). (See *American Journal of Clinical Nutrition*, May 1994, pp. 1187S-96S.)

Therapy Recommendations

Stay away from the macrobiotic diet. Children should definitely not be on it because of the threat to their growth and development. Adults are also putting themselves at risk by not getting sufficient nutrients to maintain bone and muscle tissue.

Cross-References

See "Carbohydrates," "Cruciferous Vegetables," "Fiber."

MAGNESIUM

Illnesses associated with a magnesium deficiency include diabetes, kidney disease, and hyperthyroidism. Prolonged stress, exercise, or diarrhea create additional risk. But a magnesium deficiency has not been reported in people consuming normal diets.

Magnesium depletion with or without symptoms has been reported in numerous disease states. Usually, they fall into one of six categories: inability to absorb magnesium from the gastrointestinal tract; excessive fluid and electrolyte losses; kidney dysfunction; malnutrition; alcoholism; and situations associated with special medical treatments such as nasogastric suction (involving tubes from the nose to the stomach), intragastric or intravenous feeding of mixtures deficient in magnesium.

The most prominent and consistent signs of a magnesium deficiency are nausea, muscle weakness, irritability, and mental derangements, such as hallucinations.

Basic Nutritional Therapy

The RDA for men is 350 milligrams of magnesium per day. For women the RDA is 280 milligrams, but pregnant and nursing women require additional amounts. See your physician for guidance if you are in these last two categories.

As mentioned above, magnesium deficiency may

occur for a number of reasons, including inadequate dietary intake. Even more likely is that excessive amounts of magnesium may be lost through heavy perspiration during exercise, or through the urine as a result of diuretic medications taken for high blood pressure. Various diseases, such as high blood pressure, diabetes, and heart problems, may also use up magnesium stores.

To replenish this mineral, eat magnesium-rich foods or take supplements, or both. (See "Food Sources.")

Extra Scientific Information

- In a survey done in Belgium, the mean intake for magnesium was 271 milligrams per day. This was similar to levels found in most other countries, but below the RDA value for healthy adult men (350 mg/day), and about adequate for healthy women (280 mg/day). (See *Z. Lebensm Unters Forsch*, September 1995, pp. 213-7.)
- Infant diets in the United States are likely to supply adequate amounts of magnesium for the growing child, according to a 1995 review of the scientific literature by members of the Department of Nutrition, University of California, Davis. Magnesium deficiency and toxicity are rare in infants, and are usually a consequence of hormonal abnormalities and the mother's use of large doses of magnesium. (See *Magnesium Research*, March 1995, pp. 99-105.)
- Magnesium, calcium, phosphorus, and iron are important to the support of a wide variety of body functions, such as the mineralization of bones, properly operating enzyme systems, and sustained health and growth of muscles and nerves, according to a 1995 report from the University of Massachusetts.

Most athletes appear to have adequate magnesium and phosphorus status, but those athletes on calorie-restricted diets may not take in enough magnesium. Some studies have suggested that magnesium status is indirectly related to strength improvement, as well as to reducing the incidence of muscle cramps. (See *Medical Science Sports and Exercise*, June 1995, pp. 831-43.)

- Magnesium is involved in a wide range of biological activities, including some that may protect against the development of asthma and chronic airflow obstruction, according to a 1995 study at the University of Nottingham City Hospital in Great Britain.

Scientists there examined the hypothesis that high dietary intake of magnesium is associated with better lung function and reduced wheezing. They found that increasing magnesium intake by 100 milligrams per day significantly improved respiratory functioning.

Their conclusion: Dietary magnesium intake is independently related to lung function and wheezing in the general population. Low magnesium intake may therefore be one cause of asthma and chronic obstructive airways disease. (See *Lancet*, August 6, 1994, pp. 357-62.)

- A 1994 Swedish study showed that giving doses of 365 milligrams of magnesium per day to mild and moderate hypertensive patients, who were being treated with beta-blockers, could result in a significant decrease in systolic blood pressure.
- A 1994 study at the National Hospital, Oslo, Norway, revealed a significant deficit of magnesium in many otherwise healthy elderly patients. Magnesium supplementation not only improved their magnesium status, but also helped the functioning of their kidneys. (See *Journal of the*

American College of Nutrition, February 1994, pp. 45-50.)

• Excessive intake of magnesium orally is not harmful to people with normal kidney function. But with impaired kidney (renal) function, "hypermagnesemia" can occur. Symptoms include nausea, vomiting, low blood pressure, and as the condition worsens, slow heart rates (bradycardia). Also, there may be changes in the electrocardiogram (EKG) and depression. At the most severe level of hypermagnesemia, respiratory depression, coma, and death may occur.

• Magnesium may also play a role in preventing a migraine headache. There is some evidence that it can stop a migraine headache if given at the earliest stage, and good evidence that magnesium reduces the number of migraines. (See *Environmental Nutrition*, November 1994.)

Special Food Sources, Strategies, and Facts

Rich food sources of magnesium include: cocoa and chocolate, most nuts (one cup of almonds = 380 milligrams), fish and shellfish, legumes (such as peas and lentils), kelp (one tablespoon = 100 milligrams), corn, soybean sprouts, lima beans, whole wheat muffins, taco shells, bran flakes, toasted wheat germ (one cup = 360 milligrams), brown rice, other grain and grain products, dried figs, dried pears, bananas, and dark, leafy green vegetables.

Therapy Recommendations

You should be able to get all the magnesium you need from your diet. (See "Food Sources.") But a magnesium oxide or magnesium carbonate supplement of about 50 to 100 milligrams per day is acceptable, especially if you are athletic, perspire a great deal, have hypertension and are taking medications for it, or are in one of the other higher risk groups mentioned at the beginning of this entry. It is wise to check with your physician before you go on magnesium supplements, particularly if you are taking other medications such as high blood pressure drugs.

Caution: Reports from an NIH workshop on supplements and exercise at Bethesda, Maryland, June 3-4, 1966, warned that ingestion of magnesium supplements of more than 500 milligrams per day often results in diarrhea and other gastrointestinal disturbances.

Cross-References

See "Calcium," "Electrolytes," "Heart Disease."

MEAT

Meat has received some bad press in recent years, and there is certainly a connection between the consumption of steak and pork and an increased risk of heart disease and various cancers, including cancer of the stomach, lymph glands, colon, and prostate. (See "Cross-References.")

But it's important to understand exactly what kind and quantity of meat may be bad for you personally, given your particular health history and risk status. Also, you should know the circumstances under which consuming meat may actually work to your advantage.

Basic Nutritional Therapy

First of all, growing children should usually have two to three servings of lean meat per week to get the complete amino acids, protein, and other nutrients essential for full growth and development. If your family is opposed to eating red meat, a child should be able to achieve a healthy nutritional status with daily helpings of chicken and fish, as well as a wide consumption of fruits, vegetables, and milk products.

It is possible for children to get what they need on a *very well-designed and supervised* vegetarian diet. But in my opinion, the danger is almost always too great that most children will be malnourished on a vegetarian regimen. (See "Macrobiotic Diet" entry.)

Adults whose growth and development are completed are in a lower risk category. They can usually embark on a meatless diet quite effectively, either a well-designed vegetarian program (not a macrobiotic diet), or a diet where they substitute fish and chicken for red meat.

It may be that you like steak and pork dishes, and you are adamant about not giving them up. If you are at a low risk for heart disease or cancer, eating red meat twice a week shouldn't hurt you.

There are even some circumstances when meat may play a therapeutic role in a diet. In particular, I have found that some of my patients with naturally low "good" HDL cholesterol (below about 35 mg/dl) can benefit from a prescriptive use of limited amounts of lean steak. By including two servings of lean steak twice a week (3 to 4 ounces per serving), a number of patients have succeeded in raising their HDL levels.

If you do eat red meat, you should follow these guidelines in your food preparation:

- Limit your intake to two servings per week, with about 3 to 4 ounces of meat per serving.
- Be careful about your cooking technique. Cooking meat too long and at too high a temperature will increase your risk of stomach cancer, according to a study presented in April 1996 at a meeting of the American Association for Cancer Research in Washington.

Researchers noted that red meat has been linked to heart disease because of its high saturated fat content; it has also been associated with a higher risk of colon cancer. In this study of nearly 700 healthy people and cancer patients in Nebraska, the risk of stomach cancer increased steadily with the increasing "doneness" of the meat and also with the presence of pan gravy in the servings.

The scientists conducting the study suggested that it is best to cook meat all the way through, but not so thoroughly that it is well done. Also, cook it at a relatively low temperature so that the outside of the meat doesn't turn brown or black. Because the burning process produces carcinogens, this technique of cooking is to be avoided.

- Ground meat presents a somewhat different problem. Various studies at Tufts New England Medical Center have shown that hamburger and other ground beef should be cooked all the way through to eliminate toxins and bacterial contaminants that can produce diarrhea and other health problems. This means that the inside of the ground meat should be cooked to a heat level of 165 degrees, or hot enough to eliminate all the pinkness but not to burn the meat.

I suggest that you choose lean loin cuts over ground meat because of the greater nutritional value of most steak, and also the possibility of getting a cut with a lower fat content. (See "Amino Acids," "Fat.")

Therapy Recommendations

If you have no problems with high cholesterol or blood lipids, and your doctor regards you at low risk for cancer, feel free to include two small to moderate servings of lean red meat each week (approximately 3 to 4 ounces per serving).

But be sure not to burn the steak; cook it to a "medium" done level.

To counter any fats and carcinogens in the meat, eat at least five to seven servings of vegetables and fruits every day. This will also help you keep your fiber intake at 20 to 35 grams per day.

If you have a problem with high "bad" LDL cholesterol, avoid red meat. You can eat fish and lean chicken from which you remove all visible skin and fat.

If you have low "good" HDL cholesterol but not high "bad" cholesterol, you can have two servings of lean steak (select cut) each week. (See "Basic Nutritional Therapy.")

If you have a history of cancer or are at high risk because of a family history of cancer, avoid red meat.

Cross-References

See "Amino Acids," "Atherosclerosis," "Cancer," "Cholesterol," "Fat," "Fiber," "Protein."

MEDITERRANEAN DIET

The "Mediterranean Diet," or "Mediterranean Diet Pyramid," as this program is sometimes called, focuses on food patterns typical of Crete, Greece, and southern Italy in the early 1960s. In that culture, adult life expectancy was among the highest in the world, with very low rates of coronary heart disease, certain cancers, and other diet-related chronic diseases. Also, the lifestyle of this population included regular physical activity and was associated with low rates of obesity.

Basic Nutritional Therapy

The Mediterranean Diet is characterized by an abundance of plant foods such as fruits, vegetables, breads, cereals, potatoes, beans, nuts, and seeds. Fresh fruit is the typical daily dessert, and olive oil is the principal source of fat.

Dairy products, mostly cheese and yogurt, are consumed in low to moderate amounts. Egg consumption is zero to four per week per person. Red meat is eaten in low amounts, and wine is drunk in low to moderate amounts (1-2 glasses a day), normally with meals.

Overall, the diet is low in saturated fat (no more than 7 to 8 percent of total daily calorie intake), with total fat ranging from about 25 percent to more than 40 percent of daily calories. (See a more detailed description by Dr. W. C. Willett of the Harvard School of Public Health and his co-authors in *American Journal of Clinical Nutrition*, June 1995, pp. 1402S-6S.)

People on this diet typically eat red meat only a few times a month or an average of 1 ounce per day; 4 to 6 ounces of poultry three or four times a week; and 4 to 6 ounces of fish three to seven times per week. In addition, they eat beans, nuts, or legumes every day.

As part of the total diet program, daily physical exercise is recommended. There is also the option of drinking wine in moderation on a daily basis.

My own opinion of this diet is generally positive except for the high proportion of total fat and the open-ended approach to alcohol. I would still recommend, as I have in other contexts, that total daily intake of fat amount to no more than about 20 to 30 percent of calories. Also, I have serious reservations about opening the door to greater consumption of alcohol. Although a number of studies have shown benefits of low to moderate drinking, I believe the dangers of drinking to excess outweigh these benefits. (See entries on "Alcohol" and "Wine.")

In any event, I do affirm the emphasis on fruits, vegetables, grains, and monounsaturated fats like olive oil.

Extra Scientific Information

- A 1995 study at the Universita di Milano in Italy reported an inverse relationship of breast cancer risk with intake of olive oil and other vegetable oils. In other words, the more olive oil you consume, the lower your risk. But there was no protective factor associated with butter or margarine. (See *Cancer Causes and Control*, November 1995, pp. 545-50.)
- In a study of more than 200 cases of cancer of the larynx in Milan, Italy, those who consumed high amounts of olive oil, vegetables, citrus fruits, and orange juice experienced more success in the treatment of the disease. Those who had a high intake of butter and whole milk also had a higher expectation of getting cancer.

The researchers said that their study of dietary patterns showed a 36 percent increase in survival for cancer patients whose food habits corresponded to the Mediterranean Diet. They concluded that the diet may indeed interfere with the mechanisms of cancer progression, and suggested that dietary intervention could be a means of improving survival in patients with laryngeal cancer. (See *International Journal of Cancer*, January 26, 1996, pp. 308-13.)

- It is possible that natural antioxidants in olive oil help prevent oxidation of "bad" LDL cholesterol, the major underlying cause of atherosclerosis, or clogging of the arteries. (See an Italian study reported in *Atherosclerosis*, September 1995, pp. 25-32.)
- Increased olive oil consumption was associated with significantly reduced breast cancer risk in an investigation at the Athens School of Public Health, Greece. The researchers concluded that the consumption of vegetables and fruits is inversely

associated with the risk of breast cancer. That is, the more you eat them, the more you are protected.

Also, they confirmed evidence that while olive oil consumption may reduce the risk of breast cancer, margarine intake appears to be associated with an elevated risk for the disease. (See *Journal of the National Cancer Institute*, January 18, 1995, pp. 110-6.)

Special Food Sources, Strategies, and Facts
See discussion under "Basic Nutritional Therapy."

Therapy Recommendations
Use a modified Mediterranean Diet by limiting fats to 20 to 25 percent of your total daily intake of calories. At least one-third of those fat calories should come from Mediterranean-type monounsaturated oils, such as olive oil.

Cross-References
See "Alcohol," "Atherosclerosis," "Carbohydrates," "Cholesterol," "Fat," "Fiber," "Heart Disease," "Wine."

MELATONIN
Melatonin has gained a reputation as the miracle supplement of the moment. The claims have ranged from a cure for insomnia and jet lag to antiaging and sex-enhancing properties. But, as with most such "miracles," there are as many questions as answers, as physicians and researchers examine this product more closely.

Basic Nutritional Therapy
The facts, as we currently know them, are these:
Melatonin, a hormone produced by the pineal gland in the brain, plays a role in the body's sleep cycle. It is derived

from the amino acid tryptophan and is able to influence the actions of serotonin and dopamine in the brain.

In people whose melatonin mechanism is working properly, the levels of the hormone increase rapidly in the late evening, peak after midnight, and then decrease as dawn approaches.

Older people who have trouble sleeping tend to have lower blood concentrations of melatonin. Also, the melatonin cycle can be upset when we travel rapidly from one time zone to another; hence, the motivation to use melatonin as an antidote to jet lag.

However, unless your doctor specifically prescribes this drug, I cannot recommend it for a number of reasons:

- The research still isn't solid enough for my taste. In fact, the most significant studies seem to have been with animals, not human beings.
- The best dosage has not been established. If it is used for sleep, the usual recommended dose of 2 to 3 milligrams may be far too much for many people. I know individuals who, under the supervision of their physicians, have overcome their insomnia with only 0.5 milligram.
- The quality of the drug is not regulated by the FDA. As a result, the quality of the supplement in some products is far inferior to that in others.

In one recent report on the Cable News Network (CNN), five different tablets were evaluated. While four of the five had reasonably accurate levels of melatonin as advertised, the fifth item was far off the amount indicated on the label.

- There may be unpleasant side effects, such as headaches, hangovers, or mood swings including depression.
- Even the experts recommend that many groups of

people should stay away from melatonin. These include children, pregnant or nursing women, couples trying to have a baby, mental patients, steroid users, those with serious allergies, HIV, or AIDS, and cancer patients, especially those with leukemia or other immune-related malignancies.

For the present, I suggest that you steer clear of melatonin, unless your physician prescribes and supervises its use for insomnia or jet lag.

But what about the future? The latest scientific information provides some idea about the direction recent research is pointing.

Extra Scientific Information

To understand the true promise of melatonin, consider these findings:

- A preliminary study in Italy of treatment of brain tumor patients, whose disease was given a very poor prognosis, suggests that the use of radiotherapy with melatonin may prolong survival time and improve the quality of life. (See *Oncology*, January-February 1996, pp. 43-6.)
- Used with other therapies, melatonin can improve the immune capacity of cancer patients after surgery, according to a 1995 Italian study. (See *Journal of Biological Regulation of Homeostatic Agents*, January-March 1995, pp. 31-3.)
- Melatonin, along with other therapies, may be effective in inducing regression of tumors and prolonging survival of patients with cancers of the colon and rectum. (See *Oncology*, May-June 1995, pp. 243-5.)
- Regression of tumors in patients with breast cancer may be achieved with the help of melatonin therapy.

(See *British Journal of Cancer*, April 1995, pp. 854-56.)

- Nighttime levels of melatonin were lower in patients with multiple sclerosis who were depressed than patients in a control group. (See *International Journal of Neuroscience*, February 1993, pp. 227-40.)

My observation: Manipulation of melatonin in depressed MS patients may be a worthwhile line of treatment for qualified physicians to explore with their patients.

- The presence of high melatonin levels in the blood may provide a protective effect from multiple sclerosis, while a decline in melatonin secretions may increase the risk and exacerbation of the disease. (See *International Journal of Neuroscience*, February 1993, pp. 209-25.)

My observation: Let's accelerate melatonin research with MS patients!

Special Food Sources, Strategies, and Facts

One of the most outspoken advocates of melatonin has been Dr. Russel J. Reiter of the Department of Cellular and Structural Biology, The University of Texas Health Science Center at San Antonio.

In various journal articles and other publications, he has argued that melatonin is a potent antioxidant that can scavenge the hydroxyl radical, perhaps the most powerful of all the free radicals. In this capacity, Dr. Reiter says, melatonin may be able to retard the aging process, as well as protect the central nervous system and the body's cells from free radical attack.

Also, Dr. Reiter believes that melatonin stimulates the body's production of glutathione peroxidase, which plays a part in the neutralization of free radicals. Various animal studies show that through these and other actions, melatonin can prevent cataracts and markedly reduce damage to cell DNA.

Therapy Recommendations

As you can see, melatonin does seem to have strong potential. But at the present time, the most promising possibilities seem to involve controlled scientific research or strict supervision in the context of a physician-patient relationship.

As far as private, over-the-counter use is concerned, I favor a conservative approach and recommend that you stay away from this powerful drug unless your physician prescribes it for you.

Cross-References

See "Insomnia," "Multiple Sclerosis."

MULTIPLE SCLEROSIS

There are indications that multiple sclerosis, a chronic disease of the nervous system that may lead to paralysis, an inability to walk, and other problems, can be triggered or affected by diet.

Basic Nutritional Therapy

In a study conducted at the University of Ferrara in Italy, scientists compared food consumption by patients with multiple sclerosis and healthy controls.

Among children and adolescents, they found an association between the disease and a high consumption of bread and pasta, butter, lard, legume soup, horse flesh, coffee, and tea.

They determined that adults with multiple sclerosis had a distinct dietary pattern, with an emphasis on eggs, wine, and mineral water.

The researchers concluded that some foods, consumed at certain ages, could play a causal role in the onset of multiple sclerosis. (See *Acta Neurologica*, August 1994, pp. 189-97.)

In an earlier study done at the Department of Neurology, University of Rijeka, Croatia, investigators analyzed nutritional factors that could cause multiple sclerosis in Croatia, a high-risk zone for the disease. They found that people with the disease had a high consumption of unpasteurized milk, animal fat, smoked meat, and lard.

The researchers concluded that these foods are nutritional risk factors that can influence the severity of "demyelination" in multiple sclerosis. (Demyelination involves a deterioration of the sheathing of nerves, a process characteristic of the disease.) (See *Neuroepidemiology*, 1993, pp. 234-40.)

Finally, recent research in Italy indicates that melatonin, the hormone produced by the pineal gland in the brain, can be used to relieve or treat multiple sclerosis. For more on this, see the entry "Melatonin."

Investigators from the Oregon Health Sciences University evaluated 144 multiple sclerosis patients who had followed a low saturated fat diet for 34 years. (They consumed no more than 20 grams of saturated fat per day, or the equivalent of 180 saturated fat calories.) Most of the fat they ate came from vegetable oils.

Those with minimal disability at the start of the study benefited the most, with a significantly lower death rate and a greater ability to remain physically active. (See *Lancet*, 336:37, 1990.)

In another study, MS patients with minor disabilities were treated with fish oil. They tended to have less deterioration, severity and duration of relapses with the disease than either a control group or those with more severe disabilities. (See *Journal of Neurology*, 52:18, 1989.)

Extra Scientific Information

An interesting letter from one of my patients reported a dramatic improvement of his multiple sclerosis after he took doses of nitroglycerin. Before the medication, he felt extremely fatigued and had difficulty walking. After going on regular doses of nitroglycerin, however, his energy and mobility returned.

One idea about how the nitroglycerin may have accomplished this came from an executive at the National Multiple Sclerosis Society. He suggested that while nitroglycerin has no known effect on multiple sclerosis, nitric oxide may have played a part because of its beneficial effects on the immune and nervous systems.

My conclusion: It's obviously too early to consider this approach for clinical treatment of MS, but we can hope that future scientific research will take these observations into account.

Special Food Sources, Strategies, and Facts

See the discussion under "Basic Nutritional Therapy."

Therapy Recommendations

In my opinion, a patient with multiple sclerosis would have little to lose by going on a low-fat diet and eliminating the foods mentioned under "Basic Nutritional Therapy." Many of the foods listed as possible causes or aggravators of multiple sclerosis, such as lard or other high-fat items, should not be a part of any healthy diet.

Cross-References

See "Caffeine," "Carbohydrates," "Fat," "Fiber," "Melatonin."

OBESITY

Despite the great emphasis our culture places on getting into shape, steadily increasing numbers of Americans are overweight.

According to a series of polls conducted by Louis Harris and Associates, in February of 1996, 74 percent of Americans twenty-five years old or older were overweight. In contrast, in 1983, 58 percent were overweight. The figure rose to 64 percent in 1990, 69 percent in 1994, and 71 percent in 1995.

Unfortunately, obesity is not benign. This condition, often defined as being over 20 percent of your optimum body weight (or roughly 25 to 35 pounds overweight for the average-sized person), has been implicated in a variety of diseases, including adult-onset diabetes, hypertension (high blood pressure), birth defects (including spina bifida), and certain types of cancer.

Also, being overweight is one of the three major factors that accelerate the aging process. (See the "Longevity" entry.) In a September 1995 report in the *New England Journal of Medicine*, Harvard researchers studying an extensive population of female nurses found that modestly overweight women were 60 percent more likely to die early than the thinnest women. ("Modestly overweight" was defined as a woman about 5' 5" tall, weighing between 160 and 175 pounds.)

Basic Nutritional Therapy

Some people who have chronic, genetically linked problems with obesity may have to rely on medications or even surgery to take off the extra pounds. Your physician can help you determine if you are in this category. But most people can use nutritional and lifestyle strategies to achieve their optimum weight.

The tried-and-true way to take off extra weight is simply

to take in fewer calories than you burn up. An effective way to do this is to increase the amount of fiber in your diet, because this food is relatively low in calories and tends to make you feel "full" after you have eaten a serving or two. (See the "Fiber" entry.)

As part of a high-fiber diet program, you should take in a relatively high proportion of your daily calories (at least 50 to 70 percent) as complex carbohydrates, including fruits, vegetables, especially cruciferous vegetables, and whole grain cereals and other whole grain products. (See "Carbohydrates," "Cruciferous Vegetables.")

It's been claimed that the reason Americans are fatter now than they were fifteen years ago is because obesity experts have encouraged us to eat less fat and more carbohydrates, such as pasta and bread. For example, in the book *Enter the Zone* by Barry Sears, the author claims our national weight gain is strictly the result of excess carbohydrates.

Yet the real problem, according to the National Center for Health Statistics, is still our fat intake. Surveys show that we took in an average of 81.4 grams of fat per day in the late 1970s, and 82.0 grams of fat per day in the 1980s. Also, as we are taking in 100-300 calories more per day, we are exercising less than we were in the late 1970s.

The real secret to weight loss, then, is simple: Reduce your calorie intake, or burn up more of the calories you take in, or both. (See *Nutritional Action Healthletter*, July-August 1996.)

Finally, all effective weight loss programs must be combined with regular exercise, including endurance exercise such as walking. You will not only burn up extra calories this way (walking one mile uses up about 100 calories), but you will also increase your lean muscle mass as you take off the fat. Lean muscle automatically uses up more calories than does fat. Regular exercise is an essential component in establishing a lower-weight lifestyle that will help you avoid putting back on the pounds you have lost.

The most accurate way to determine your level of obesity is to measure body fat. Many fitness centers perform body fat measurements by using calipers that lightly pinch key parts of the body. The measurements are then plugged into an equation that tells your percent of body fat. In more sophisticated centers, such as our Cooper Clinic in Dallas, underwater weighing techniques are also used.

In general, here are some guidelines about what your weight should be:

For women: Those younger than forty should have less than 22 percent body fat. Those forty and over should have no more than 26 percent body fat.

For men: Those under forty should have less than 19 percent body fat. Those forty and over should have no more than 20.5 percent body fat.

For more precise age-related body fat recommendations, see the appendix of my *Aerobics Program for Total Well-Being* (Bantam, 1983).

Another important risk factor involves the location of the extra fat on the body. There has been a trend in recent years to highlight the waist-to-hip ratio. In other words, the more fat a person has on the waist and chest in relation to the hips and thighs, the higher the risk for a variety of diseases, including:

- High blood pressure
- High triglycerides (a lipid in the blood that is associated with heart disease)
- Coronary heart disease
- Low levels of "good" HDL cholesterol
- Diabetes

Since there is no established way to do spot reductions, the best strategy for eliminating your upper body fat is to go on a general weight-reduction program to slim down the entire body. (The waist-hip ratio in men should be less than 0.85, and in women less than 0.75.)

Extra Scientific Information

- In a 1995 study at the Mayo Clinic, Rochester, Minnesota, obese women with mild to moderate hypertension achieved weight losses that resulted in significant improvements in blood pressure, lowering of total cholesterol, lowering of "bad" LDL cholesterol, and lowering of triglycerides. (See *Obesity Research*, September 1995, pp. 217S-22S.)
- Weight loss can improve ovulation, pregnancy outcome, self-esteem, and endocrine function for women who are infertile and overweight, according to research at the University of Adelaide, Australia. (See *Human Reproduction*, October 1995, pp. 2705-12.)
- Swiss researchers compared two diets in a 1996 report. One had 15 percent carbohydrates (along with 32 percent protein and 53 percent fat). The other consisted of 45 percent carbohydrates (plus 29 percent protein and 26 percent fat). The investigation showed no difference in weight loss on the two diets.

The conclusion: It was energy intake, not nutrient composition, that determined weight loss in response to low-energy diets over a short period of time. (See *American Journal of Clinical Nutrition*, February 1996, pp. 174-8.)

- Weight loss of eight kilograms (about 17.5 pounds) in moderately obese individuals has led to significant decreases in blood pressure, and stabilization of plasma glucose and insulin concentrations. (See

American Journal of Hypertension, November 1995, pp. 1967-71.)

Special Food Sources, Strategies, and Facts

See discussion under "Basic Nutritional Therapy."

Therapy Recommendations

See my suggestions under "Basic Nutritional Therapy."

Cross-References

See "Atherosclerosis," "Cancers," "Carbohydrates," "Cruciferous Vegetables," "Fiber," "Heart Disease," "Longevity."

OLESTRA

Olestra is a fat substitute approved by the U.S. Food and Drug Administration in January 1996 and designed to be used in potato chips, crackers, and other snack foods.

The good news is that foods containing olestra (trade name Olean), which was developed and marketed by Procter & Gamble, have a dramatically lower calorie content than the regular versions. For example, a typical serving of regular potato chips contains 10 grams of fat and 150 calories, while chips with olestra have 0 grams of fat and only 70 calories.

The bad news is that olestra can have side effects in some people, including abdominal cramping, gas, and loose stools. In one study, half of the subjects developed diarrhea after eating three ounces of potato chips made with olestra. Other studies have found that even one ounce of chips caused diarrhea and cramps in some people. Also, there is a chemical action that inhibits the absorption of some vitamins and other nutrients. In particular, problems have arisen in the absorption of vitamins A, D, E, K, and the carotenoids, the nutrients found in carrots and sweet potatoes.

Basic Nutritional Therapy

Even though more than 150 long- and short-term studies show no harm from olestra, I still am reluctant about giving a wholehearted go-ahead to my patients and readers. Also, I am concerned about the possible blocking effect in the body on various vitamins and other nutrients, and whether the added supplementation will be adequate or effective.

However, if no-fat snack foods are part of your diet, the chances are you won't be able to avoid olestra in the future. My best advice would be to read the labels of any snack foods or other no-fat items, and try to limit your intake of olestra-containing foods to no more than one serving per day. Also, be sure that you take your antioxidant cocktail to replenish important nutrients, particularly beta-carotene, that may be lost through the action of the olestra. (See Chapter 4.)

My preference is always to focus on the natural diet foods, such as low-fat or no-fat fruits and vegetables or fiber. (See "Carbohydrates," "Cruciferous Vegetables," "Fiber," "Obesity.")

Extra Scientific Information

- Fats and oils account for 38 percent of the total calories in the diets of Western populations and especially in the U.S. Because of the high calorie content of fats, efforts are being made to find fat substitutes, such as olestra (sucrose polyester). According to researchers at the Department of Food Science and Technology, University of Georgia, these "designer fats" may be the trend of the future to produce medical lipids that do not occur normally in nature. (See *Critical Review of Food Sciences and Nutrition*, September 1995, pp. 405-30.)

- In a study conducted at Western General Hospital in Edinburgh, healthy participants took 24 grams of olestra per day for thirty-six days. They did not experience interference with the normal intestinal fermentation of dietary fiber or any significant alterations of bacteria in the gut. (See *European Journal of Clinical Nutrition*, September 1995, pp. 627-39.)
- In animal studies, heating olestra before it was consumed did not change the absorption qualities of the fat substitute. (See *Fundamental Applied Toxicology*, February 1995, pp. 229-37.)
- Olestra was found not to be toxic or carcinogenic, even when it represented 10 percent of an animal diet and was fed to the animals for a period of two years, according to a Procter & Gamble study. (See *Food Chemical Toxicology*, September 1994, pp. 789-98.)
- The use of olestra in amounts of up to 30 grams in a 45-gram fat meal does not significantly alter the gastrointestinal transit time of food in healthy people, a Mayo Clinic (Rochester) study reported in 1993. (See *Digest of Disease Science*, June 1993, pp. 1009-14.)

Olestra can deplete the body of fat-soluble vitamins, including A, D, E, and K, as well as carotenoids such as beta-carotene. In one study, eating sixteen olestra potato chips a day for eight weeks reduced blood carotenoids by 50 percent. In another study, six chips a day lowered beta-carotene levels by 20 percent.

To combat these problems, Olean (olestra) will be fortified with vitamins A, D, E, and K, but not with carotenoids. If there are questions in anyone's mind that deficiencies of beta-carotene are related to lung cancer and heart disease, we may soon find out definitely as olestra is used more extensively.

Therapy Recommendations

See my comments under "Basic Nutritional Therapy." And, here is another suggestion to protect yourself: If you consume olestra-containing foods and notice any of the symptoms mentioned in the introduction to this entry, stop eating those foods immediately. There is a good chance that you have a sensitivity to olestra and should not include it in your food program.

Cross-References

See "Fat," "Fiber," "Obesity."

OSTEOPOROSIS

Osteoporosis, the bone-thinning disease that results in frequent fractures, afflicts an estimated 25 million Americans. The disease is particularly a problem for older women, who may develop low bone-mineral density, low bone-mineral content, and a loss of bone quality.

Dietary factors generally regarded as important in maintaining bone quality include overcoming deficiencies of calcium and vitamin D, and increasing intake of protein and phosphates. Also, minerals such as magnesium and potassium, and other nutrients such as flavonoids may be important in maintaining bone health. (See *British Journal of Biomedical Science*, December 1994, pp. 358-70. Also, consult my book *Preventing Osteoporosis*, Bantam, 1989.)

Basic Nutritional Therapy

The best dietary and lifestyle approach to preventing osteoporosis, or countering the destruction of bones once the disease has begun, can be summed up this way:

1. Take in at least 1,000 to 1,500 milligrams of calcium per day. Your first line of defense should be foods high in calcium, such as dairy products, canned sardines, and turnip greens. But most likely, you will have to use supplements to achieve this level of intake. (See "Calcium" entry.)

2. Engage in weight-bearing exercise three to four times a week. This means walking, jogging, doing calisthenics, and using light weights. Putting weight on the bones tends to stimulate bone growth. (For exercises and other information, see my *Preventing Osteoporosis*, Bantam, 1989.)

Caution: If you already have osteoporosis, exercise may cause fractures. Be sure to check with your physician before you embark on any exercise program.

3. Consider hormone replacement therapy (HRT). This therapy, which involves taking regular doses of estrogen and progestin, may be appropriate if you have had your ovaries removed, are going through menopause, or have already passed through menopause. (See "Hormones" entry.)

Here are a couple of guidelines to keep in mind if you are thinking about HRT:

- Women should have their bone density checked by age forty. If the actual density is lower than about 85 percent of the expected density for the patient's age, the physician may prescribe bone-building medications or other special therapy.
- If your bones are sufficiently healthy at age forty, you will probably be advised by your physician to focus on a bone-building diet with plenty of calcium and exercise until you reach menopause.

Another bone-density test should be performed at menopause. If the recorded density is still above 85 percent of expected density, you may be able to continue to rely on calcium intake and exercise to keep your bones strong. Also, if your only problem is menopausal symptoms, such as hot flushes, you may want to try including foods containing "phytoestrogens" in your diet, such as wild yams and soybeans. (See the "Hormones" entry.)

Many women do go on HRT at this stage of life, either because of the threat of osteoporosis or for other reasons, such as risk of heart disease or severe menopausal symptoms. (Again, see the "Hormones" entry.) Your physician will have to advise you on this matter.

Extra Scientific Information

- The abundance of vitamin K in bones suggests an important function for this nutrient, but the precise role of vitamin K remains to be determined.

Blood concentrations of vitamin K are reduced in older people and those with osteoporotic fractures. So, vitamin K insufficiency has a possible role in osteoporosis, but more research is required on this topic. (See *Journal of Nutrition*, July 1995, pp. 1812-21.)

- For breast-feeding mothers, bone loss or depletion of bone mass caused by breast-feeding can be reduced through adequate maternal nutrition, a prolonged period of weaning, and adequate spacing of childbirth. (See *International Journal of Gynecology and Obstetrics*, December 1994, pp. S11-21.)
- Osteoporosis-related bone fractures are a significant cause of mortality and morbidity, with women being particularly affected, according to a 1994 report from the University of Portsmouth in England.

An adequate supply of calcium is essential to attain maximum bone mass, and adult intakes below about 500 milligrams per day may predispose a person to low bone mass. It is also important to correct chronically low intakes of vitamin D, and possibly magnesium, boron, fluoride, vitamins K, B_{12}, B_6, and folic acid—all of which may predispose a person to osteoporosis. *Note:* Exercise acts as a catalyst with calcium in maintaining or building new bone.

Similarly, chronically high intakes of protein, sodium chloride, alcohol, and caffeine may negatively affect bone health. (See *British Journal of Biomedical Science,* September 1994, pp. 228-40.)

- Pernicious anemia has been identified as a risk factor in osteoporosis and in fractures of the femur, forearm, and vertebrae.
- Administration of high doses of vitamin K to postmenopausal women for 24 and 48 weeks significantly increased bone mass, compared to women treated with a placebo. (See *Journal of Bone and Mineral Research*, 7 [Suppl. 1] S122, 1992.)
- Forty asymptomatic, postmenopausal women (average age sixty-one years, and at least five years without menstruation), were studied after doing 45 minutes of weight-bearing exercise, twice weekly for 50 weeks. Their activity resulted in a highly significant increase over a control group in three bodily areas: hip and back bone density, total body mineral content, and muscle mass. Both groups took 800 mg of supplemental calcium daily, but no hormone replacement therapy (HRT) was used. (See *Journal of the American Medical Association*, December 28, 1994.)

Special Food Sources, Strategies, and Facts

See the listings under "Calcium" and "Hormones" entries, and also food tables and descriptions in my book *Preventing Osteoporosis.*

Therapy Recommendations

See the comments under "Basic Nutritional Therapy," and also the recommendations in the "Calcium" and "Hormones" entries.

Cross-References

See "Bioflavonoids," "Caffeine," "Calcium," "Vitamin D," "Hormones," "Vitamin K."

PANTOTHENIC ACID

Pantothenic acid, which once was referred to as vitamin B_5, has developed a reputation as an "antistress" vitamin because of its involvement in the production of adrenaline (or epinephrine), which is secreted by the adrenal glands during times of fear, excitement, or other stress. Also, this nutrient assists in the production of coenzyme A, a key player in the body's metabolism.

Generally speaking, there is no need to worry about suffering from a deficiency of this vitamin because many foods contain it, and only 4 to 7 milligrams a day have been set as an estimated safe and adequate daily intake.

Basic Nutritional Therapy

Although there is usually no toxicity associated with pantothenic acid (for an exception, see "Extra Scientific Information"), it is still best to stick to foods containing this vitamin rather than relying on supplements. (See "Food Sources.")

Still, taking small doses of 20 to 50 milligrams as part of a multivitamin capsule should do no harm and may even have benefits for some people, mitigating the effects of stress (fatigue or nervousness), or even relieving acne. (See "Extra Scientific Information.")

Extra Scientific Information

- Liberal use of pantothenic acid may be able to bring about relief from severe acne, according to a report from the Department of General Surgery in the Hong Kong Central Hospital. (See *Medical Hypotheses*, June 1995, pp. 490-2.)
- Supplementation with pantothenic acid and ascorbic acid (vitamin C) may help wounds to heal, according to a report from Hospices Civils, Strasbourg, France, published in *European Surgery Research*, 1995, pp. 158-66. This study involved forty-nine patients undergoing surgery for removal of tattoos. For twenty-one days, they received a daily supplementation of 1 gram of vitamin C and 0.2 gram of pantothenic acid.
- Pantothenic acid is more "bioavailable" (more readily available to the human body) in finely ground maize bran than in coarsely ground maize bran or finely ground corn bran. (See *Plant Foods in Human Nutrition*, January 1993, pp. 87-95.)
- A patient with dermatitis (inflammation or irritation of the skin) was found to be allergic to dexpanthenon, a derivative of pantothenic acid. (See *Contact Dermatitis*, February 1993, pp. 81-3.)

Special Food Sources, Strategies, and Facts

Rich food sources of pantothenic acid include: chuck roast, various beef steak cuts, lamb leg and chops, Canadian bacon, ham, veal, wild game, cashews, hazelnuts, peanuts, sunflower seeds, chicken dark meat, duck, turkey, abalone, lobster, salmon, trout, corn, mushrooms, pinto beans, whole baked potato, tomato paste, toasted wheat germ, pumpkin pie, buckwheat flour, soy flour, wheat bran, bulgur, brown rice, wild rice, skim milk, nonfat dry milk, eggnog, plain skim yogurt, avocados, dates, pomegranates.

Therapy Recommendations

It's best to focus on getting pantothenic acid through your diet. But, if you have serious problems with stress, including stress-related symptoms like fatigue and anxiety, you might try a moderate supplemental dose of this vitamin, up to about 50 milligrams a day. This amount has never been shown to do any harm, and who knows? You might be one of those people who responds quite positively to the nutrient!

Cross-References

See "Wounds, Healing."

PERNICIOUS ANEMIA

Pernicious anemia involves an inability of the body to absorb vitamin B_{12}. The only way this vitamin can go through the wall of the small intestine is to be helped along by a stomach secretion known as the "intrinsic factor." If this factor is absent, as sometimes happens with aging, pernicious anemia may result. The problem is one of inadequate absorption, not poor intake.

Some of the symptoms of pernicious anemia are gastritis or inflammation of the stomach lining, inflammation of the tip of the tongue, numbness and tingling in the hands and feet, diminution of the ability to sense vibrations and body position, poor muscular coordination, poor memory, and hallucinations.

Basic Nutritional Therapy

Those diagnosed with pernicious anemia are treated with B_{12} injections of 50 to 100 milligrams, three times a week for several weeks. Then they are given the injections once a month for the rest of their lives. Oral supplementation can be given in very large doses, but this method is expensive and seldom used.

Care must be taken in determining the cause of the anemia. Folic acid, given in the presence of a vitamin B_{12} deficiency, may correct the anemia to some extent. But it may not correct some signs of the vitamin deficiency, such as progressive neurological symptoms. Furthermore, if this condition isn't detected early, the neurological changes can become irreversible.

Extra Scientific Information

- Pernicious anemia has recently been recognized as a risk factor for osteoporosis and fractures. For two years, scientists at the University of Michigan followed a patient with severe osteoporosis, multiple fractures of the vertebrae, and pernicious anemia. The patient showed dramatic response to treatment with vitamin B_{12} injections and the medication "cyclic etidronate." He also took 1,500 mg of calcium and 400 IUs of vitamin D daily. In fact, bone density measurements showed a 15 percent increase in the lumbar spine, a 17 percent increase in the hip, and a 79 percent increase in the femoral neck.

The researchers concluded that osteoporosis associated with pernicious anemia may be markedly improved by vitamin B_{12} replacement and cyclic etidronate therapy. (See *Metabolism*, April 1994, pp. 468-9.)

Therapy Recommendations

Vitamin B_{12} injections are the accepted treatment for those with pernicious anemia, including those patients with both pernicious anemia and osteoporosis. Obviously, these diseases must be treated by qualified physicians.

Cross-References

See "Vitamin B$_{12}$," "Folic Acid," "Osteoporosis."

PROTEIN

Proteins, carbohydrates, and fats are the three basic food categories that most people must consume daily to stay healthy and energetic. Protein plays a key role in the growth and maintenance of muscle and other body tissues. (See "Carbohydrates" and "Fats" entries.)

Basic Nutritional Therapy

The discussion under the entry "Amino Acids" contains most of what you need to know about protein in your diet, but here is a recap, along with some special facts not included elsewhere:

First, remember that the average, healthy person should take in 10 to 20 percent of daily calories in the form of protein. (See "Special Food Sources" and "Therapy Recommendations.") You can learn how to calculate these percentages by turning to the "Amino Acids" section.

Note: Some diets, such as those for patients with kidney disease, are "protein restrictive." They may specify low amounts of protein, say, about a half gram of protein a day per kilogram of body weight. A high-protein diet, which might be designed for those who need to build lean body mass (muscle), could require a daily intake of 2 grams of protein per kilogram of body weight.

On the low-protein diet, a 150-pound person would consume about 35 to 40 grams of protein per day, or about 140 calories. On a 2,000-calorie diet, this amount would translate into only about 7 percent of total calories. In contrast, the high-protein diet (2 grams per kilogram) would total 130 to 135 grams, or about 530 calories. That would be over 25 percent of the calories on a 2,000-calorie diet.

Finally, let me offer a few observations on protein supplements:

If protein supplements are taken in moderate amounts, they appear to be safe for most people. In fact, there are many anecdotal accounts, and some scientific support for claims that they contribute to the building of muscle tissue and endurance. (See "Extra Scientific Information" and also the "Amino Acids," "Creatine Supplements" entries.)

In addition to the studies already detailed in the entry on creatine supplements, several recent scientific and anecdotal reports have indicated some success in animal and human studies with supplements based on beta-hydroxy-beta-methylbutyrate. This is a protein product also known as "HMB."

HMB, which is derived from a breakdown of the amino acid leucine, reportedly has put extra meat on livestock and more muscle on athletes. One unpublished study presented at an experimental biology conference in Washington, D.C., in 1996, and reported by the Associated Press, claimed that college athletes taking 3 grams of an HMB supplement daily had a 3.1 percent lean muscle mass gain. This contrasted with a 1.94 percent gain in athletes who did not take the supplement.

Also, the HMB users were reported to have lost 7.3 percent of their body fat. The non-HMB group, on the other hand, lost only 2.2 percent of their body fat. (See "Extra Scientific Information" for more details.)

Unfortunately, at this point the scientific evidence on such supplements is scanty, and so I cannot recommend them. If you are an athlete who needs to put on muscle mass, they may be worth a try, provided that you undergo regular blood and urine tests and regular medical check-ups.

Extra Scientific Information

- Feeding beta-hydroxy-beta-methylbutyrate (HMB) to sows at a level of 2 grams per day resulted in an increase in fat percentage in the sow's milk and in the pig's overall physical performance, according to a 1994 Iowa State University study. (See *Journal of Animal Science*, September 1994, pp. 2331-7.)
- Feeding HMB to steers tended to increase the ratio of intramuscular fat (as compared with subcutaneous fat) and also the lipid content of the muscles, researchers at Oklahoma State University reported in 1994. (See *Journal of Animal Science*, August 1994, pp. 1927-35.)
- Chickens given doses of HMB experienced greater longevity, and the incidence of sudden death syndrome in the broilers decreased, according to Iowa State University investigators. (See *Poultry Science*, January 1994, pp. 137-55.)
- Dietary protein restriction may help a patient overcome the body's rejection of a kidney transplant. The mechanism may be due partly to the suppression of the kidney's renin-angiotensin system, according to scientists from the Department of Medicine, University of Minnesota. (See *Kidney International Supplement*, December 1995, pp. S102-6.)
- Supplementary protein nutrients can improve human biochemical and nutritional health, and also the functioning of the stomach lining, according to Japanese scientists at the Hamamatsu Medical Center. (See *Advanced Peritoneal Dialysis*, 1993, pp. 80-6.)
- HIV patients with stable body weight took whey-based protein powder over a three-month period in a 1993 study conducted at Montreal General

Hospital, Quebec. They gained between two and seven kilograms (about 4.5 to 16 pounds), and they also experienced an elevation of a natural body antioxidant, glutathione (GSH). (See *Clinical Investigations in Medicine*, June 1993, pp. 204-9.)

Special Food Sources, Strategies, and Facts

See food listings under the "Amino Acids" entry.

Here are some other suggestions for increasing your protein. Each of the indicated servings of the following foods contains about 5 to 6 grams of protein:

> One ounce of fish
> One ounce of chicken without the skin
> One ounce of lean tenderloin or sirloin steak
> One ounce of lean pork or ham
> One ounce of low-fat cheese
> One large whole egg
> One-fifth cup of mature cooked soybeans
> One cup of fortified bran flakes
> One-fifth cup of toasted wheat germ

Therapy Recommendations

Design your diet so that 10 to 20 percent of your daily calories comes from protein. Children who are still growing need protein intake on the higher end of this range. Also, athletes who are trying to build muscle and strength should go for higher amounts.

As you design your diet, pay particular attention to the amino acids contained in the foods you choose. (See "Amino Acids.")

Athletes and others particularly concerned about keeping up their energy and endurance levels should emphasize complex carbohydrates, though protein also plays an important role in their diets. Specifically, those needing a higher carbohydrate level should try to take in 60 to 70 percent of their daily calories through complex carbohydrates such as fruits, vegetables, and whole grain products like pasta. (See the discussion on carbohydrate loading under "Carbohydrates.")

Cross-References

See "Amino Acids," "Carbohydrates," "Creatine Supplements," "Fat."

PYCNOGENOL

Pycnogenol, a commercial mixture of bioflavonoids derived from plant materials, operates as an antioxidant, much like vitamins E and C. For many health food enthusiasts, this substance is the supplement of the moment; but we lack scientific study on the impact of Pycnogenol on humans.

Basic Nutritional Therapy

In animal studies, Pycnogenol and related substances known as "proanthocyanidins" and "anthocyanins," have demonstrated the ability to:

- Increase immunity.
- Increase the contraction force of muscles.
- Suppress tumors.

Also, there are anecdotal accounts that this supplement can benefit those with chronic fatigue, psoriasis, skin problems, varicose veins, arthritis, and a variety of other complaints.

Undoubtedly, some of these improvements are the result of the placebo effect, a physical response to a belief that the medication will work. But some of the results, especially those related to the antioxidant qualities of the drug, may have a chemical basis as well.

In any event, more scientific data will be required before we can know exactly what Pycnogenol can do in the human body. As a result, I cannot recommend it at this time.

Extra Scientific Information

- Pycnogenol is the trade name of a commercial mixture of bioflavonoids (catechins, phenolic acid, proan, thocyanidins) that exhibits antioxidative activity, according to researchers doing animal studies at the University of Arizona. In their 1996 report in *Life Science* (pp. 87-96), they found that natural killer cell cytotoxicity, which is a key to the immune function, was increased with Pycnogenol treatment.
- A Pycnogenol-related extract, proanthocyanidin, which is derived from the bark of pine trees found on the French coast, was tested on nerve and muscle regeneration in mice by Italian scientists in 1995. They found an increase in the contraction force of muscles and concluded that proanthocyanidin exerts a nutritional effect on muscle. (See *Boll Soc. Ital. Biol. Sper.*, July-August 1995, pp. 227-34.)
- Proanthocyanidins are also found in grape seeds.
- Anthocyanins, bioflavonoids extracted from flower petals, were found to have the ability to suppress tumor cells. (See *Cancer Investigations*, 1995, pp. 590-4.)
- In a 1995 British study, researchers examined the antioxidant power of anthocyanin-related flavonoids, which are found in fruit, vegetables, tea, and wine. They determined that in fighting destructive free radicals, these extracts are four times more powerful as antioxidants than a type of vitamin E. (See *Free Radical Research*, April 1995, pp. 375-83.)

Special Food Sources, Strategies, and Facts
See "Basic Nutritional Therapy."

Therapy Recommendations
See "Basic Nutritional Therapy."

Cross-References
See Chapter 4 on antioxidant therapy.

SALT (SODIUM CHLORIDE)

Salt, which is 40 percent sodium and 60 percent chloride, is an essential mineral in the human body because it helps regulate the water balance and plays a role in various nerve, muscle, and cell functions. Also, iodized salt is one of the richest dietary sources of iodine, which is important in maintaining the thyroid function. (See "Iodine.")

But almost no one has to worry about getting enough salt! The average American takes in an estimated 3,000 to 6,000 milligrams of sodium per day, an amount equal to 7,500 to 15,000 milligrams of salt! Yet the body usually requires less than 1,000 milligrams per day to operate properly.

The main challenge, especially for those with high blood pressure, is to cut back on salt, not add it to the diet. (See "High Blood Pressure.")

Basic Nutritional Therapy

In addition to its mineral functions, salt is also an electrolyte the body may lose through heavy perspiration, diarrhea, vomiting, or other loss of fluids. Contrary to some popular notions, salt tablets are not recommended as a means to correct this loss. Either plain water or diluted electrolyte-based drinks are preferred. (See the "Electrolytes" entry.)

People who have high blood pressure should severely restrict their salt intake. (See discussion under "Special Food Sources.") Also, I suggest that even those with no blood pressure problems should still limit their intake of sodium to no more than 3,000 to 3,500 milligrams per day (the equivalent of 7,500 to 8,750 milligrams of table salt).

One reason for this restriction is that a number of non-hypertensive problems have been linked to high salt intake, including loss of calcium and bone deterioration, stroke, enlargement of the heart, kidney stones, and asthma. (See "Extra Scientific Information.")

Extra Scientific Information

- About 60 percent of people with hypertension respond to a high salt intake with a rise in pressure, and to salt restriction with a fall in pressure and reduction in the need for antihypertensive medications, according to a 1995 review article from the Department of Physiology, Uniformed Services University of the Health Sciences, Bethesda, Maryland.

How does salt retention raise blood pressure? One possibility is that salt retention causes water retention, which releases a digitalis-like substance that increases the contraction of the heart and blood vessels. Another possible explanation is that the sodium itself penetrates the smooth muscle cells of the vessels, causing them to contract.

Finally, there is evidence that salt-sensitive hypertension can be relieved through increased potassium and calcium intakes, perhaps in part because these minerals increase the excretion of salt through the urine. (See *Journal of the American College of Nutrition*, October 1995, pp. 428-38.)

- Salt intake not only plays an important role in determining blood pressure, it has also been shown to have other negative effects on health, independent of blood pressure, according to a 1995 review article by researchers from St. George's Hospital Medical School in London. These nonhypertensive problems associated with salt intake include: stroke mortality, left ventricular hypertrophy (enlargement of the left ventricle of the heart), cerebral artery disease, and death from asthma. Also, reducing sodium intake reduces calcium excretion, which may cut down on bone demineralization and hip fractures. (See *Clinical Experiments in Pharmacology and Physiology*, March 1995, pp. 180-4.)
- Reduction of salt in the diet may be a useful strategy to decrease the risk of forming calcium-containing kidney stones, according to investigators at Washington State University. (See *Nutrition Review*, May 1995, pp. 131-9.)

Special Food Sources, Strategies, and Facts

Most salt in our diet comes in through processed foods. For example, many ice creams and commercial desserts are quite high in salt content.

Here are some typical sodium values in different foods (reprinted with permission from *The Balancing Act* by G. Kostas and K. Rojohn, copyright 1989):

    1 medium apple—1 mg
    1/8 of a frozen apple pie—482 mg
    1 slice of bread—130 mg
    1 tablespoon of margarine—150 mg
    3 ounces of baked chicken—86 mg
    3 ounces of fried, fast-food chicken—500 mg
    1 tablespoon of soy sauce—1,330 mg
    1 teaspoon of salt—2,130 mg

3 ounces of tuna in water—372 mg
1 ounce cheddar cheese—174 mg
1 cup canned tomato soup—970 mg

When calculating the amount of salt vs. sodium in your food, remember that salt contains roughly 40 percent sodium and 60 percent sodium chloride. So, you multiply the number of grams of salt by 0.40 to get the grams of sodium. Or, you can multiply the number of grams of sodium in an item of food by 2.5 to get the salt content.

Therapy Recommendations

I usually advise my patients to avoid adding table salt to food if they are at any risk for high blood pressure. Patients concerned about their blood pressure should be on a low-sodium diet (2,000 milligrams or less daily). Non-hypertensive individuals may consume a little more, although I recommend that everyone stay below about 3,000 to 3,500 milligrams of sodium per day.

The salt that is naturally in meats and other foods, as well as salt seasonings often used in the cooking process, supplies more than enough of this mineral. Consequently, there is really no need for anyone, hypertensive or non-hypertensive, to add more at the table. If you have a particularly high need for the kind of taste that accompanies salt on food, try a salt substitute or another seasoning. Increasing numbers of them are appearing on pharmacy and supermarket shelves.

Cross-References

See "Calcium," "Electrolytes," "High Blood Pressure," "Iodine."

SELENIUM

The mineral selenium is an antioxidant that is available through the diet, especially in shellfish and certain grains cultivated in selenium-rich soil. (See "Special Food Sources.")

It is also a structural element of the human enzyme glutathione peroxidase. In this capacity, it protects the natural antioxidant glutathione, which is found in human cells and serves as part of the body's internal defenses against free radical damage.

In addition, selenium works hand in hand with vitamins C, E, and beta-carotene to fight oxidation in human cells, though large doses of vitamin C can interfere with the absorption of selenium. Through this mechanism it may reduce the risk of a number of diseases, including asthma, heart disease, and cancers of the stomach and esophagus. Low blood selenium is involved in the development of macular degeneration, poor color vision, and impaired "blue-cone" response (a specialized eye test). *Note:* The eye probably has higher free radical activity than any other organ, and several eye diseases are undoubtedly the result of excess free radical production.

Basic Nutritional Therapy

The scientific evidence for selenium is still at a relatively early stage, and so I continue to consider selenium supplementation as optional. (See Chapter 4.) This means that I regard it as an acceptable, but optional, supplement when taken in doses of 50 to 100 micrograms per day. (The RDA is lower: 70 mcg per day for men, and 55 mcg per day for women.)

It is not clear at this point that more than 100 micrograms of selenium per day would be helpful to your health. Furthermore, if you move beyond a total intake of about 400 micrograms per day (supplements plus food sources), you could approach the range of negative or toxic effects. Various studies have shown that excess selenium can stimulate tumor growth and produce side effects like loss of hair, brittle fingernails, nausea, vomiting, diarrhea, nerve disease, irritability, or fatigue. (See "Extra Scientific Information.")

Extra Scientific Information

- Supplementation of the diet with antioxidative vitamins and selenium increases the protection of low-density lipoproteins (LDL or "bad" cholesterol) in human blood against the oxidation process. Oxidation of LDL contributes to the formation of plaque in blood vessels and heart disease, according to a 1994 Finnish report.

In this study, otherwise healthy male smokers, ages thirty to fifty-eight, took the following supplements daily for a three-month period: 100 micrograms of organic selenium, 400 milligrams of slow-release ascorbic acid (vitamin C), 200 milligrams of natural vitamin E, and 30 milligrams of beta-carotene. As a result of this treatment, the oxidation process in their blood decreased significantly. (See *European Journal of Clinical Nutrition*, September 1994, pp. 633-42.)

- The ability of high-selenium garlic to protect against tumors in animals is primarily dependent on the increased intake of selenium provided by the garlic, researchers from the Roswell Park Cancer Institute in Buffalo, New York, reported in 1995. (See *Carcinogenesis*, November 1995, pp. 2649-52.)
- The selenium status of a group of Russians studied by the National Public Health Institute in Helsinki, Finland, was fairly good, thanks to the high selenium content of imported wheat. (See *Biological Trace Elements Research*, March 1994, pp. 277-85.)
- A vegetarian diet fails to provide a sufficient supply of essential antioxidant trace elements like zinc,

copper, and especially selenium, according to a
study by the Institute of Preventive and Clinical
Medicine, Bratislava, Slovak Republic. (See
Biological Trace Elements Research, October 1995,
pp. 13-24.)

• Chinese researchers studied patients with symptoms
of selenium toxicity, including broken hair strands
or various levels of nail damage. They determined
that the maximum safe daily dietary selenium intake
should be 400 micrograms. (See *Journal of Trace
Elements and Electrolytes in Health and Disease*,
December 1994, pp. 159-65.)

• In an investigation by the University of Verona, Italy,
of residents in a northern Italian village, aging was
associated with a progressive decrease in selenium
status. (See *American Journal of Clinical Nutrition*,
May 1995, pp. 1172-3.)

• Both selenium and conjugated linoleic acid are powerful agents in suppressing animal tumors. (See
Cancer Research, April 1, 1994, 7 Supplement, pp.
157S-9S.)

• A substantial body of evidence indicates a lack of
any appreciable effect of selenium intake on the risk
of breast cancer in humans, according to Harvard
School of Public Health scientists M. Garland, W. C.
Willett, and colleagues. (See *Journal of the American
College of Nutrition*, August 1993, pp. 400-11.)

Special Food Sources, Strategies, and Facts

Good food sources of selenium include the following
(approximate micrograms of the mineral are indicated):
brown rice (80 micrograms per cup), enriched white rice
(65 mcg per cup), whole wheat flour (80 mcg per cup),
orange juice (15 mcg per cup), wheat bran (35 mcg per cup),
beef liver (50 mcg per 4 ounces), round steak (170 mcg per

pound), half breast of chicken (20 mcg), one chicken drumstick (14 mcg), vinegar (13 mcg per tablespoon), clams (100 mcg in 9 large), cod (37 mcg in 3 ounces), lobster (95 mcg in 3 ounces), oysters (45 mcg in 6 medium), scallops (70 mcg in 3 ounces), shrimp (180 mcg in 3 ounces).

Therapy Recommendations

Rely on the above food sources for your selenium. Taking supplements of 50 to 100 micrograms of selenium per day is an option, but don't go above a total of about 400 micrograms per day, including dietary intake plus supplements.

Cross-References

See "Vitamin A," "Vitamin C," "Vitamin E," Chapter 4.

SICKLE-CELL ANEMIA

Sickle-cell anemia is a disease of the blood characterized by a sickle-type shape of the red blood cells. Dark-skinned people, or those of African background, are most susceptible to this disease, which may trigger strokes as a result of excessive clotting of the blood.

A nutritional link to this disease is a deficiency of vitamin B_{12} (cobalamin). In a study conducted at King Saud University, Riyadh, Saudi Arabia, scientists examined the levels of vitamin B_{12} in patients with severe sickle-cell disease, as compared with controls. Complete blood counts, iron studies, and vitamin B_{12} levels were measured.

The results showed that 43.5 percent of the sickle-cell patients had serum vitamin B_{12} levels below normal. Furthermore, the patients with low B_{12} levels achieved a significant improvement in their symptoms after being treated with intramuscular injections of 1 milligram (1,000 micrograms) of vitamin B_{12} once a week for twelve weeks.

The researchers concluded that many patients with severe sickle-cell disease may suffer from unrecognized vitamin B_{12} deficiency. (See *Journal of Internal Medicine*, June 1995, pp. 551-5.)

Basic Nutritional Therapy

An important feature of nutritional therapy in sickle-cell anemia is to avoid excessive iron storage. The diet should be designed to be low in iron by eliminating such foods as liver and iron-fortified cereals. In addition, the diet should be low in fat (less than 30 percent of total calories).

Requirements for the water-soluble vitamins (C, A, E, and K) are high because of the continual need to replace large numbers of red blood cells. Supplemental zinc may also be of value (20-30 mg per day) since zinc is lost when red blood cells are destroyed.

The diet should be high in folate (400-600 mcg per day). The reason: The increased production of red blood cells increases the body's folic acid requirements. Administration of a folate supplement (400 mcg per day) is also recommended.

Cross-References

See "Vitamin B_{12}."

SOYBEANS AND SOY PRODUCTS

For centuries, soy products have been widely used in Asia for nutrition as well as for medicinal purposes. More recently, their benefits have become known in the West as scientific studies have analyzed the effects of these products on health.

Reports in different scientific journals have associated soybean products with lower risk of many health problems, including heart and vessel disease, various cancers, kidney disease, and osteoporosis (the thinning and deterioration of the bones that occur with aging).

Basic Nutritional Therapy

Soybean protein is "complete" protein. This means that for complete absorption by the body, it doesn't require the consumption of animal protein as found in dairy products or meats. As a result, soy products can play a major role in a balanced vegetarian diet. (See "Amino Acids" and "Protein" entries.)

Various scientific studies have shown that regular consumption of soy foods may contribute to the relatively low rates of breast, colon, and prostate cancers in such countries as China and Japan. The reason for this effect is thought to be the presence of "anticarcinogens," or anti-cancer agents such as vitamin E and phytoestrogens, in soy. Some investigations suggest that there may also be an antioxidative factor in soy products, which counters the destructive work of free radicals. Free radicals are increasingly being implicated in cancer, heart disease, and a host of other health problems. (See Chapter 4 for more on free radicals and antioxidants.)

In this vein, a number of studies have linked soy consumption to lower levels of "bad" LDL cholesterol in the bloodstream. This association establishes soy products as a good means to reduce the risk of vessel disease and heart attacks. (See "Extra Scientific Information.")

Also, soy products contain hormone-like substances that display weak estrogen-like activity and thus reduce the symptoms of menopause. (See the "Hormones" entry.)

Extra Scientific Information

- In two-thirds of the animal studies on the effect of soy foods, specifically the chemical genistein, which is present in soy, the risk of cancer was reduced significantly. (See *Journal of Nutrition*, March 1995, pp. 777S-83S.)

- A wide variety of scientific studies show that isoflavonoids, which are hormonelike, plant-produced "phytoestrogens" found in soybean products, are natural cancer-protective compounds. (See *Journal of Nutrition*, March 1995, pp. 757S-70S.)
- Although noting that more research needs to be done, scientists from Northwestern University suggest that greater incorporation of soybean products into the human diet may be a safe and effective means of reducing cancer risk. (See *Journal of Nutrition*, March 1995, pp. 751S-6S.)
- Here is more on specific cancers:

There is much evidence to suggest that diets containing large amounts of soybean products are associated with overall low cancer mortality rates for cancers of the colon, breast, and prostate, according to a review article produced at the University of Pennsylvania in 1995. The authors say that supplementation of human diets with certain soybean products, especially those which have been shown to suppress carcinogenesis in animals, could markedly reduce human cancer mortality rates. (See *Journal of Nutrition*, March 1995, pp. 733S-43S.)

- In an investigation at the Division of Foods and Nutrition, University of Illinois at Champaign-Urbana, researchers found that consumption of 25 grams of soybean protein per day for four weeks was associated with lower total cholesterol concentrations in individuals with high cholesterol levels. (See *Journal of Nutrition*, February 1994, pp. 213-22.)
- The type of cooking method used with soybean products has an influence on risk of cancers of the

stomach, according to a 1995 study from Hanyang University College of Medicine, Seoul, Korea.

Specifically, cooking soybean paste stew, hot pepper-soybean stew, and other broiled and salted dishes increased the risk of stomach cancer. But low-salt dishes, such as tofu (soybean curd), actually decreased the risk of stomach cancer.

The researchers concluded that heavy salt consumption, and cooking methods like broiling and salting foods heavily, seem to play a major role in stomach cancer among Koreans. (See *International Journal of Epidemiology*, February 1995, pp. 33-41.)

- Dietary therapy should be the first step in the treatment of high blood lipids, including cholesterol, according to researchers from Washington University School of Medicine in St. Louis, Missouri.

Furthermore, the use of adjuncts to the diet, such as soluble fibers, garlic, and soy protein, may allow lipid concentrations to be lowered without the use of drugs. For example, soy protein, when incorporated into a low-fat diet, can reduce total cholesterol and "bad" LDL cholesterol concentrations.

The authors pointed out that even though tofu and soy milk are available in many stores, American consumers are often unaware of their presence and use. Consequently, it is necessary to provide more readily available packaged products, recipes, and cookbooks to spread the word about soy. (See *Journal of Nutrition*, March 1995, pp. 675S-8S.)

- Soybeans have played an integral part in Asian culture for centuries, both as a food and as a medicine, according to a 1995 review article in the *Journal of Nutrition*. In the West, soybeans are best known for their protein content. Only recently have they been recognized for prevention and treatment of cancer, heart disease, osteoporosis, and kidney disease.

The existing database on the health effects of soy food intake is quite extensive and clearly warrants greater recognition by the research and clinical communities. In addition, soy foods such as tofu, soy milk, and soy concentrates and flours can be incorporated into the American diet with relative ease. (See *Journal of Nutrition*, March 1995, pp. 567S-69S.)

- Soy foods may contribute to the relatively low rates of breast, colon, and prostate cancers in China and Japan, according to a 1994 report from the National Cancer Institute in Bethesda, Maryland.

In addition, soybeans are a dietary source of the isoflavone genistein, which possesses weak estrogenic activity. Genistein has also been shown in animal studies to have the power to suppress growth of a wide range of cancer cells. (See *Nutrition and Cancer*, 1994, pp. 113-31.)

- In a study by the Tufts University School of Medicine in Boston, the estrogen activity of phyto-estrogens was examined in five different foods: tofu (soybean curd), a commercially produced soy drink, and three soy-based formulas.

The researchers found that tofu contained the highest amounts of isoflavones (estrogenlike substances). The soy drink contained lesser amounts, and the soy-based formulas had no estrogenic activity. (See *Journal of the American Dietetic Association*, July 1994, pp. 739-43.)

Special Food Sources, Strategies, and Facts

Soybeans and soybean products are packed with good nutrition. For example, in one cup of cooked soybeans, you get about 240 calories, including 20 grams of protein (80 calories), 20 grams of carbohydrates (80 calories), 9 grams of fat (81 calories), and 3 grams of fiber.

Cooked soybeans have an abundance of calcium (88 milligrams), phosphorus (211 milligrams), potassium (443 milligrams), and a variety of amino acids. Furthermore, soybeans and soy products are a good source of phytoestrogens, which can provide a woman with weak natural hormones that may decrease the symptoms of menopause. (See "Hormones" entry.)

The fats in soy products are overwhelmingly unsaturated. As you know from the discussion under the "Cholesterol" and "Fat" entries, saturated fats are linked to higher levels of "bad" LDL cholesterol. In contrast, unsaturated fats have a protective effect against atherosclerosis and heart disease.

Other good sources of soy include soybean sprouts, soybean milk, soy flour, and tofu (soybean curd).

Caution: Soy products should not be cooked by broiling or with heavy salting because these methods of food preparation have been associated with increased stomach cancer risk. (See "Extra Scientific Information.")

Therapy Recommendations

Soybean products should be a part of most food programs, with at least two or three servings a week and preferably more. Their link to a lower risk of cancer, heart disease, osteoporosis, and other diseases makes them one of the best forms of nutritional therapy.

One possible exception: Women taking hormone replacement therapy to reduce the symptoms or health risks of menopause, or who are on estrogen and progestin for other reasons, should check with their physicians before including any of the foods containing phytoestrogens in their diet. (See the "Hormones" entry.)

Cross-References

See "Amino Acids," "Calcium," "Cancers," "Cholesterol Regulation," "Folic Acid," "Fiber," "Heart Disease," "Hormones," "Iron," "Protein."

WATER

Water, even more than food, is necessary to sustain life. It's been estimated that the average person can exist only four to six days without the intake of any fluids. In contrast, people have survived many weeks without food.

For optimum health, much more than a minimal intake of water is necessary, as is evident in the following discussion.

Basic Nutritional Therapy

Everyone should drink the equivalent of at least eight 8-ounce glasses of water per day. While it is best actually to drink those eight glasses of water as water, it is also possible to bring part of this fluid into your system by drinking natural fruit juices, such as orange or grapefruit juice.

You may even be able to reach your daily water quota by eating extra helpings of fruits and vegetables with a generous water content. But this approach can be difficult to monitor, because the amount of water in different fruits and vegetables varies greatly. A good way to keep track of the level of fluids in your system is to check the color and amount of your urine. Clear, frequent urination indicates that you have plenty of water in your system. Dark, yellow urine, on the other hand, may be a sign of too little water.

If you tend to perspire a great deal or you are particularly active in sports, you should drink even more than eight glasses per day. For example, a registered dietitian with the International Bottled Water Association, Felicia L. Busch, has suggested these amounts for one hour of exercise at different intensities: (See *Tennis* magazine, June 1996):

- If you weigh 115 pounds, you should take in 9 (8-ounce) cups a day if you do one hour of light exercise (such as playing doubles); 9.5 cups a day for moderate exercise (such as tennis singles); and 10 cups a day for strenuous exercise (such as tournament tennis play).
- If you weigh 150 pounds, you should take in 9 cups a day for light exercise; 10 cups a day for moderate exercise; and 11.5 cups a day for strenuous exercise.
- If you weigh 200 pounds, you should take in 9.5 cups a day for light exercise; 11 cups a day for moderate exercise; and 13.25 cups a day for strenuous exercise.

What are the symptoms of drinking too little water?

Aside from the color and frequency of the urine, dehydration, even to a slight extent, can greatly impair mental acuity and physical performance, and the victim may not even be aware of the problem. The signals of a mild lack of body fluids include lower physical performance levels, fatigue, an inability to concentrate, or irritability. (See "Extra Scientific Information.") These dehydration signals may begin to appear when you have drunk too little water in the course of a particular day, or after a bout of the flu accompanied by diarrhea or vomiting.

More extreme cases of dehydration may involve dizziness, heat exhaustion, or heat stroke, which can lead to a loss of consciousness and even death.

A note on serious dehydration: The symptoms of heat exhaustion are profuse sweating, clamminess of the skin, light-headedness, and sometimes loss of consciousness. The best first-aid treatment is to have the person sit down in a cool, shaded place and drink plenty of water or diluted electrolyte-based drink. (See "Electrolytes.")

The symptoms of heat stroke are a failure to perspire, unusually hot skin, and possible loss of consciousness. The best first-aid response is to cool the entire body quickly by using ice, cold water, or cold packs. Also, because this condition is an emergency, you should call an ambulance service or physician. It is possible to die from a heat stroke.

Extra Scientific Information

- A 1995 study, conducted at the Ribstein Center for Research and Sport Medicine Sciences, Wingate Institute, Netanya, Israel, examined the effect of water restriction on basketball players. The researchers divided ten healthy male players into teams of two, and had each team participate in two "two-on-two" full-court basketball games for a forty-minute period. Water consumption was permitted in one game but not in the other.

The players began each game with plenty of water in their bodies, and they performed jump tests prior to each game, at halftime, and also immediately after each game. In addition, the performance of the players was measured by calculating field goal percentages and free throw percentages during each half of each game.

The researchers found no significant differences in anaerobic (short-burst, sprinting) power or jumping ability between the groups who were given water during the games and those who were not. But they did find a 19 percent difference in anaerobic power in favor of the water groups over the no-water groups *after* the games. Also, they found an 8.1 percent decrease in field goal percentage in the no-water groups when first-half performance was compared with second-half performance.

Though noting that the changes did not rise to the

level of statistical significance, the scientists did say their findings suggested that high intensity, moderate duration exercise, when combined with fluid restriction, might be detrimental to performance. (See *International Journal of Sports Medicine*, May 1995, pp. 214-8.)

Special Food Sources, Strategies, and Facts

In most parts of the United States, tap water is usually as pure or purer than bottled water. But concerns are constantly being raised about the quality of water in certain areas, including some large cities. In one recent report, several public health groups, including the Centers for Disease Control and Prevention, warned about the presence in tap water of a potentially deadly parasite called "Cryptosporidium parvum." Initial symptoms may include diarrhea, cramps, fever, nausea, and vomiting. This parasite is a particular threat to those with low levels of immunity, such as AIDS patients.

To prevent problems from this parasite, those in threatened areas have been advised by public health experts to boil tap water, use a water filter that will eliminate particles less than one micron in diameter, or drink bottled water.

Whether or not you have a known problem with this parasite, it's wise to monitor reports in your area about the quality of drinking water. Then, if an alarm is sounded, you can drink bottled water until the danger has passed.

Therapy Recommendations

See "Basic Nutritional Therapy."

Cross-References

See "Carbohydrates," "Electrolytes."

WINE

St. Paul recommended to his protégé, Timothy, "No longer drink only water, but use a little wine for your stomach's sake and your frequent infirmities" (1 Tim. 5:23 NKJV).

This medicinal use of wine has a long history and has found support in recent scientific studies. (See "Extra Scientific Information.") But the potential for abuse of alcohol has caused me to suggest that my patients seek other ways to get the benefits that wine may provide.

Basic Nutritional Therapy

I do not recommend wine for nutritional therapy because there is far too much danger that it will be used to excess and create more health problems than it solves. Still, there is evidence that low to moderate amounts can provide a number of benefits, including these:

- Protection for travelers who are exposed to strange microbes and parasites in foreign food.
- Antioxidant activity to fight off free radicals that can contribute to atherosclerosis and heart disease.
- Anticoagulant activity that can help prevent the development of blood clots.

But wine definitely has its special drawbacks. One potential problem is that some people develop migraine headaches after drinking it. (See "Extra Scientific Information.")

Extra Scientific Information

- Red and white wines were tested by U.S. Army researchers to determine their effect on suspensions of potentially harmful organisms like salmonella, shigella, and Escherichia coli.

The investigators found that undiluted wine was effective in reducing the viable organisms by 1 million to 10 million colonies after twenty to thirty minutes. They concluded that the antibacterial property of wine is largely responsible for wine's reputation as a digestive aid. (See *BMJ*, December 23-30, 1995, pp. 1657-60.)

- A component of red wine called "resveratrol" has an antiaggregating (anticlotting) ability with blood platelets, according to research done at the Institute of Anatomy, University of Milan. (See *International Journal of Tissue Reactions*, 1995, pp. 1-3.) *Note:* Concord grape juice actually contains more resveratrol than most wines.
- The "French paradox," a term coined in recent medical research, refers to the very low incidence of ischemic heart disease and the low mortality rates from heart disease in France, despite the fact that saturated fat intakes, serum cholesterol, blood pressure, and smoking habits are certainly not ideal.

Scientists at the University of Wales College of Medicine have concluded that the French custom of drinking wine with the meal may confer protection against some of the adverse effects of the food. In particular, researchers noted that the relative immunity of the French to ischemic heart disease has been attributed to their high alcohol consumption and their intake of antioxidant vitamins, both of which are supplied by their wine. (See *Journal of Research in Social Health*, August 1995, pp. 217-9.)

- A 1994 study of twenty healthy Israeli males compared the health effects of red and white wines.

Half of the subjects received 400 milliliters of red wine (with 11 percent alcohol content) for two weeks. (This amounts to a little less than one pint, or a little more than one and one-half glasses of wine per day.) The other half of the group was given the same amount of white wine.

The red wine, but not the white, resulted in an 11 percent increase in plasma triglyceride concentration after one week and 26 percent after two weeks. Total cholesterol and "bad" LDL cholesterol did not change.

But the most impressive effect of the study, according to the researchers, was a significant increase in "good" HDL cholesterol (26 percent higher) among the participants who took the red wine. There was no such increase with the white wine.

The scientists concluded that the major effect of red wine consumption, which amounted to about 40 grams of alcohol per day for a period of two weeks, was a significant increase in plasma HDL levels. They said that this may contribute to the reduced risk for cardiovascular diseases observed in red-wine drinkers. (See *Annals of Nutritional Metabolism*, 1994, pp. 287-94.)

- The dietary causes of migraine headaches remain controversial, according to scientists at Queen Charlotte's and Chelsea Hospital in London. But some of the recently described pharmacological properties of red wine may trigger the sequence of events leading to migraine headaches. (See *Cephalagia*, April 1995, pp. 101-3.)
- Researchers at Princess Margaret Migraine Clinic, Charing Cross Hospital, London, questioned 577 patients, of whom 429 had migraine headaches. Of these, 16.5 percent reported their headaches were precipitated by cheese or chocolate; 18.4 percent reported sensitivity to all alcoholic drinks; 11.8 percent were sensitive to red but not white wine; and 28 percent reported that beer caused their headaches.

The scientists concluded that cheese, chocolate, and red wine sensitivity are closely related and more likely to be involved in migraines than in chronic, tension headaches. (See *Headache*, June 1995, pp. 355-7.)

- In 1995 Israeli researchers reported that consumption of red wine with meals reduces the susceptibility of human plasma and "bad" LDL cholesterol to lipid peroxidation. Oxidation of LDL is a major factor in atherosclerosis and heart disease.

The scientists concluded that some "phenolic" substances that exist in red wine, but not in white wine, are absorbed into the bloodstream, bind to plasma LDL, and may be responsible for the antioxidant properties of red wine. (See *American Journal of Clinical Nutrition*, March 1995, pp. 549-54.)

- The content of phenolic compounds in red wine is due to the incorporation of the red grape skins into the fermenting grape juice during wine production. When white wine is produced, only the fermented juice is used. Since grape skins are the primary source of phenolic compounds, white wine has a low percentage of these natural antioxidants, which scavenge free radicals and reduce their ability to oxidize lipids (blood fats). (See *Nutrition Review*, 51:185, 1993.)
- Investigators at the Department of Pathology, University of Birmingham, United Kingdom, compared the antioxidative effect on human blood of red wine, white wine, and high doses of vitamin C. The participants consumed 300 milliliters of red wine (about one glass), or the same amount of white wine, or 1,000 milligrams of vitamin C.

Those who drank the red wine increased the antioxidant capacity of their blood by 18 percent after one hour and by 11 percent after two hours. The white wine was less effective, producing increases of 4 percent and 7 percent respectively. But the vitamin C users had the strongest antioxidant response of all: 22 percent after one hour and 29 percent after two hours. (See *Clinical Chemistry*, January 1995, pp. 32-5.)

Why bother with wine at all for antioxidant activity if vitamin C produces a superior response?

Special Food Sources, Strategies, and Facts

Taken in low to moderate amounts, red wine seems to have more health benefits than white wine. (See "Extra Scientific Information.")

Therapy Recommendations

I do not recommend alcohol as a form of nutritional therapy. See my comments in the "Alcohol" entry.

Cross-References

See "Alcohol," "Atherosclerosis," "Cholesterol Regulation," "Headaches," "Heart Disease."

WOUNDS, HEALING

It is generally accepted in the medical community that in the different phases of the wound-healing process, proteins, carbohydrates, fats, vitamins, and minerals play key roles.

For example, there is evidence that in the tissue repair process that occurs after surgery, appropriate nutritional interventions by health professionals can enhance the potential for optimal wound healing. (See *Compendium*, February 1995, pp. 200, 202-4, 206-8.)

Basic Nutritional Therapy

Although overall balanced nutrition is the starting point for successful healing of wounds, the most recent research has also placed an emphasis on the role and intake of certain specific nutrients. These include vitamin A, zinc, vitamin C, vitamin E, the various B vitamins, iron, and the amino acid arginine. (For foods and supplements containing these nutrients, see "Cross-References.")

Extra Scientific Information

- Improved nutrition can improve the outlook for wound healing after dental surgery, according to researchers at the College of Nursing and Health Sciences, University of Texas at El Paso. (See *Compendium*, February 1995, pp. 200-8.)
- Proper nutrition in presurgical patients can enhance wound healing and decrease the cost of postsurgical medical care, according to the authors of a review article produced at the California College of Podiatric Medicine in San Francisco. Research in this area usually focuses on the role of protein, vitamin A, zinc, vitamin C, vitamin E, and iron. (See *Journal of the American Podiatric Medical Association*, September 1994, pp. 456-62.)
- Contrary to the preceding position, the author of another review article, from the Brown University School of Medicine, Rhode Island Hospital, concluded that there is no support in objective data for the idea that malnutrition increases the risk of wound-related complications.

The author also said that there is no support for the position that dietary intervention, through either a general food program or supplements, can improve or accelerate the wound-healing response. (See *JPEN Journal of*

Parenteral and Enteral Nutrition, July-August 1994, pp. 367-76.)

- Supplementation with protein and vitamins, specifically the amino acid arginine and vitamins A, B, and C, provides optimum nutrient support of the healing wound, reported scientists at Shriners Burns Institute, Galveston, Texas. (See *New Horizons*, May 1994, pp. 202-14.)
- Malnutrition causes an array of metabolic alterations that affect wound healing, according to a March 1993 article in the *Journal of Vascular Nursing* (pp. 12-8).

This report says that several key nutrients play specific roles in wound healing:

- Vitamin C is essential for the synthesis of collagen (connective tissue).
- Vitamin A enhances epithelization, the process by which a raw area is covered over with new skin.
- Zinc is necessary for cell mitosis (cell division) and cell proliferation.

- An animal study by the Department of Environmental Science at Hokuriku University, Kanazawa, Japan, showed that zinc can promote the appearance of cells in a wounded area. Also, the number of cells in the wounded area was significantly increased by zinc. (See *Research Communications in Molecular Pathology and Pharmacology*, August 1995, pp. 189-98.)
- Zinc is an important element in wound healing; in particular, it speeds the healing of gastric ulcers, according to animal studies performed by Japanese scientists from Osaka City University Medical School. In a report in the June 1995 issue of *Digest of*

Disease and Science (pp. 1340-4), they concluded that zinc is crucial for healing gastric ulcers, especially at the early stage of the disease.

Special Food Sources, Strategies, and Facts

See the listings for foods that may hasten and enhance healing under the entries listed in "Cross-References."

Therapy Recommendations

The best preparation for healing *before* you suffer a wound is to eat a solid diet consisting of my recommended percentages of carbohydrates, protein, and fats. (See entries for "Amino Acids," "Carbohydrates," "Fat," and "Protein.")

After a wound has been inflicted, you *may* experience more effective and quicker healing if you weight your nutrition in favor of zinc, vitamin C, vitamin A, the B vitamins, vitamin E, and the amino acid arginine. (See "Cross-References.")

Cross-References

See "Vitamin A," "Vitamin B," "Amino Acids," "Vitamin C," "Vitamin E," "Protein," "Zinc."

ZINC

Only about 2 to 3 grams of zinc are present in the human body, with about 30 percent of the mineral involved with bone tissue. Zinc, which is present in and indispensable to all forms of life, is essential for normal pregnancies, growth, and transmission of our genetic material. It is also required as an enzyme component in the eyes, liver, kidneys, muscles, skin, testes, and other organs. Virtually all cells contain zinc, but the highest concentrations are in bones, the prostate gland, and the eyes.

Zinc deficiencies, on the other hand, have been linked to infertility, spontaneous abortions, malformations of the fetus, premature and overdue births, infant deaths, later growth problems, and a host of other difficulties, including impaired immune response, abnormal taste, and abnormal night vision. In addition, too little zinc may result in delayed healing of wounds.

However, there is a delicate balance. Just as too little zinc may be disastrous, too much can pose serious dangers to health. Zinc toxicity can result in stomach upsets, diarrhea, vomiting, kidney problems, and even death. An excess of zinc may also result in a deficiency of copper in the body, which leads to anemia.

Basic Nutritional Therapy

The RDA for zinc is 15 milligrams per day for adult men and 12 milligrams for adult women, but many people take in much less than this. Also, those on vegetarian or high-fiber diets may lose much of the zinc they consume, because it is "bound" by the fiber and washed out of the body through the intestines.

On the other hand, those who try to increase their intake through supplements may get into trouble. For example, taking supplements of 100 milligrams per day or more may bring on toxicity or zinc poisoning, as described in the introduction to this entry.

I recommend that you take in your zinc through zinc-rich foods, such as those mentioned under "Special Food Sources" below. Use zinc supplements only under the guidance of a qualified physician.

As a result of a study conducted at Dartmouth College a few years ago, zinc lozenges have been recommended to lessen the severity and shorten the duration of colds. But the zinc in those lozenges was different from what is marketed today.

Nearly all commercial lozenges contain flavoring agents that literally tie up the zinc, in contrast to the original product used at Dartmouth, which allowed the zinc to be released into the saliva. If future studies confirm the Dartmouth results, scientists may have found something that can make colds less miserable. But for now, it's too early to recommend zinc-containing lozenges, even though they may be produced like those in the original Dartmouth study.

Extra Scientific Information

- Low dietary zinc intake (64 to 87 percent of the recommended dietary allowance) was not associated with reduced height in children with epilepsy in a University of California study. (See *American Journal of Clinical Nutrition*, December 1993, pp. 858-61.)

- A study at the Universita Degli Studi, Ferrara, Italy, noted that zinc deficits are frequently found in the elderly (generally, those seventy years of age or older) and may cause a reduction in cellular immunity. This makes older people susceptible to more infections and increased morbidity (disease) and mortality (death).

A low-zinc condition is particularly a problem for surgery patients and those undergoing parenteral (intravenously injected) nutrition, according to the authors. The study recommends an average daily allowance of 15 milligrams of zinc for elderly people. (See *Minerva Medicine*, June 1995, pp. 275-8.)

- A 1995 study at the University of Wisconsin Medical School reported that levels and sources of zinc intake in 1976-80 were higher than in more recent national surveys. The investigators said this suggested that overall zinc intakes may be declining. Those with the lowest levels of consumption include women, older adults, blacks, and people with lower levels of education and higher levels of poverty. (See *Journal of the American College of Nutrition*, August 1995, pp. 349-57.)

- Symptoms of zinc deficiency in a breast-fed, premature male infant included diarrhea, irritability, and a skin eruption. But after seven weeks of zinc supplementation, the child's disease was cured. (See *Australian Journal of Dermatology*, August 1995, pp. 157-9.)
- Infants can absorb the zinc in breast milk more effectively than that in cow's milk or formula. This is a significant distinction because zinc is very important for the proper growth of children.

While lactating, mothers should consume 19 milligrams of zinc daily during the first six months and 16 milligrams daily during the second six months. Also, pregnant and nursing mothers should increase their intake of seafood, lean meat, nuts, legumes, and whole grain products, which are high in zinc.

- Adult men who adopt cholesterol-lowering diets, involving an intake of approximately 30 grams of fiber per day, do not appear to be at risk for zinc deficiency. (See *Journal of the American Dietetic Association*, November 1995, pp. 1274-9.)
- In a study by the U.S. Department of Agriculture's Grand Forks Human Nutrition Research Center, North Dakota, researchers tested the zinc absorption status of fourteen women ages fifty-one to seventy. They found that those on a high-meat diet (including lean beef, chicken, ham, and tuna) enjoyed high levels of zinc absorption and retention.

They concluded that high meat consumption increases zinc retention without compromising calcium status. (See *American Journal of Clinical Nutrition*, September 1995, 621-32.)

- The increased maternal need for zinc must be met through an increased dietary intake or adjustments by the body to produce more zinc (such as release of zinc from the bones). (See *Analyst*, March 1995, pp. 895-7.)

- A premature infant fed exclusively by breast displayed severe zinc deficiency symptoms, such as erosive skin changes and loss of hair. Also, he suffered from irritability and a failure to thrive. The German researchers concluded that a diet of breast milk can, in rare circumstances, cause insufficient zinc intake and result in severe zinc deficiency. Therapy consists of oral zinc supplementation. (See *European Journal of Pediatrics*, January 1995, pp. 71-5.)

- Avoidance of red meat by premenopausal women increases the risk of iron and zinc deficiencies, according to a report from the University of Texas Medical Branch, Galveston. (See *Journal of Laboratory and Clinical Medicine*, December 1994, pp. 852-61.)

- A study of vegetarians in India revealed that zinc absorption is enhanced by foods that contain hemicellulose (a fiber component of various fruits and vegetables, which may be soluble or insoluble), milk protein, niacin, and cereal protein.

Nutrients that inhibit zinc absorption are primarily fiber and phytate. Phytate, a nonnutrient component of plant seeds, occurs in the outer husks of grains (especially in oatmeal), legumes, and seeds. Most dietary phytate comes from seeds such as cereal grains, but problems of phytate interference with zinc tend to be more a concern in developing nations than in the United States.

How much zinc actually gets into your body from the food you eat? The rate of zinc absorption from dietary sources varies from 15 to 40 percent of the amount of the mineral in a given food product. This rate is based upon a person's zinc status: If there is a zinc deficiency, more is absorbed from food. (See *Annals of Nutritional Metabolism*, 1994, pp. 13-9.)

- Zinc intake should be routinely assessed in anorexia nervosa patients who are vegetarians, and zinc supplementation of their diets should be considered. (See *International Journal of Eating Disorders*, March 1993, pp. 229-33.)
- Supplemental zinc, ranging from 17 to 50 milligrams per day, can block the healthy rise of "good" HDL cholesterol that normally accompanies exercise. Furthermore, excessive intake of zinc supplements (160 milligrams per day) can actually decrease blood levels of this "good" cholesterol. (This information comes from a presentation by Dr. Henry C. Lukaski, of the U.S. Department of Agriculture, at a June 3-4, 1996, workshop on exercise and supplements, sponsored by the NIH at Bethesda, Maryland.)
- Macular degeneration of the eye, a slow decay of the retina, is the leading cause of blindness in Americans over sixty-five years of age. Yet a diet rich in zinc may lower this risk. Therefore, older people are encouraged to supplement their diets with zinc.

Unfortunately, however, the effective dose, 100 milligrams per day, is much larger than the RDA of 15 milligrams per day. Taking such a large amount of zinc every day has been found to cause a number of problems, including: nausea, vomiting, diarrhea, stomach pain, lethargy, and fatigue. Consequently, some patients find they have to use lower, less effective doses, or they have to rely primarily on their food for zinc.

In any event, it's essential to exercise caution with larger doses. Taking up to 150 milligrams per day can affect the cholesterol metabolism and may accelerate the development of atherosclerosis. (See *Environmental Nutrition*, March 1992.)

Special Food Sources, Strategies, and Facts

Foods that contain relatively high amounts of zinc include the following:

Toasted wheat germ (1/4 cup = 8 milligrams); chuck roast (3.5 ounces = 7.8 milligrams); lean ground beef (3.5 ounces = 5.2 milligrams); various steak cuts (3.5 ounces = 4.4-5.5 milligrams); Brazil nuts (1 ounce = 1.3 milligrams); dry, roasted cashews (1 ounce = 1.6 milligrams); dry, roasted pecans (1 ounce = 1.3 milligrams); dry, roasted peanuts (1 ounce = 0.58 milligram); sesame seeds (1 ounce = 2.03 milligrams); crab (3 ounces = 5 milligrams); oysters (6 medium = an incredible 76 milligrams!); boiled black-eyed peas (1 cup = 2.2 milligrams); boiled garbanzos (1/2 cup = 1.3 milligrams).

Therapy Recommendations

Get your zinc from foods such as those listed above. Stay away from supplements unless your physician directs you to use them.

Cross-References

See "Fiber," "Wounds, Healing."

Chapter 7

Advanced Nutritional Therapy in a Nutshell

In the foregoing pages, I trust I have answered many of your questions about diet, supplements, herbs, and a variety of other subjects relating to the nutritional side of preventive medicine.

But there is one thing that does continue to bother me: As I suggest or recommend certain supplements or herbal remedies, I worry that some people may elect to treat all their symptoms herbally, or with "home remedies." This is a dangerous practice that may prevent or delay the use of proven, effective, conventional drug treatments or medical procedures.

This risk is accentuated by the lack of training and knowledge of most people in the new nutritional area of medicine. As a result, I have continually advised the reader throughout this book to consult with his or her physician before embarking on an "alternative medicine" approach.

At a minimum, your doctor should be informed about what you want to do. A personal physician is the only one who knows whether a planned treatment or preventive program is appropriate, can be used safely, and will not cause side effects or interactions with other medications. So make your physician an integral part of your preventive medicine team!

Notwithstanding these words of caution, I remain convinced that the next major breakthroughs in medicine will be in nutrition or nutrition-related fields. Specifically, I expect scientific research to show us in much greater detail how your personal health program can be adjusted and fine-tuned to deal with such issues as:

• How free radicals cause disease;
• The use of antioxidants to prevent or treat various diseases;
• The role of folic acid and homocysteines in preventing and treating atherosclerosis and heart disease;
• The use of supplements to help athletes build up their bodies and improve their performances *safely*;
• The scientific application of traditional herbal remedies; and
• The exciting potential of phytoestrogens, those plant-derived hormones that may be used to treat the symptoms of menopause and a variety of other problems.

A great deal of research certainly remains to be done. Yet enough is now known for me to recommend unequivocally that *most* people (with the exceptions noted in the text) should be consuming certain vitamins and minerals in significantly larger amounts than the Recommended Dietary Allowances (RDAs). In a nutshell, the most important of these include:

• Vitamin E. (See Chapter 4 and the alphabetical entry "Vitamin E.")
• Vitamin C. (See Chapter 4 and the "Vitamin C" entry.)

- Beta-carotene. (See Chapter 4 and the "Vitamin A" entry.)
- Folic acid. (See Chapters 2 and 3.)
- Calcium. (See the "Calcium" entry.)
- Vitamins B_6 and B_{12}. (See these entries in the alphabetical section of this book.)

Whenever possible, these items should be obtained through your daily diet. For example, you should be able to get enough beta-carotene quite easily with a well-designed food program. Other nutrients, especially one like vitamin E, will require supplementation.

Obviously, this list is not exhaustive. Some people with special health problems or concerns may be as much in need of other nutrients as those mentioned above. For example, someone with a cholesterol imbalance may be directed by a physician to take high doses of niacin (vitamin B_3).

But it's safe to say that everyone's nutritional program should at least begin with a consideration of the above items. These constitute the foundation of an Advanced Nutritional Therapy program.

On the whole, I am quite optimistic about the prospects for Advanced Nutritional Therapies. It seems clear that the future of medicine is moving slowly but definitely away from a strict emphasis on disease treatment, and toward the prevention of disease. And as I've said earlier, nutrition is the first among equals in an effective preventive medicine program.

A major reason for this change of emphasis is a growing awareness on the part of the American public. They are learning that what I have been saying for years is really true: "It is cheaper, and much more enjoyable to maintain good health than it is to regain health once it is lost."

Index

Index

Farquharson, Graham, 54-55
fat(s), 216-18
  atherosclerosis and, 105
  calories, 218
  hypertension and, 243
  ketogenic diet and, 269-71
  measurement of body, 297
  multiple sclerosis and, 292-94
  obesity and, 295-99
  olestra substitute, 299-302
fatigue, 219-21
  iron and, 263
  pantothenic acid and, 308
  pycnogenol and, 314
  vitamin B$_2$ and, 111, 112
feverfew, 236
ferritin, 97, 266-67
fertility, 39
fiber, insoluble, 221-23
  constipation and, 178, 179
  diarrhea and, 204
  diverticulitis and, 208-9
  hypertension and, 243-44
  obesity and, 296
fiber, soluble, 223-25
  constipation and, 178, 179
  diarrhea and, 204
  diverticulitis and, 208-9
  obesity and, 296
fish
  deepwater, 164
  oil, 199, 257, 293
  flaxseed, 253-44, 255
folate. See folic acid
folic acid
  benefits of, 10, 14-20, 225-26
  deficiency, 13, 17, 203, 205
  requirements, 15-16
  sources of, 14, 20-22
  therapy, 32-36, 309, 324
food
  cured/pickled/smoked, 143
  hormones in, 143
  intolerances, 79-85, 102-3
  nutrients, 59-60
free radicals
  antioxidants and, 37-38
  bioflavonoids and, 123-24, 315
  coenzyme Q10 and, 169, 172
  exercise and, 51-56
  ginkgo biloba and, 238
  homocysteines and, 28, 30
  iron and, 263

measuring, 39-40
melatonin and, 291
selenium and, 320
vitamin C and, 128
wine and, 334, 337
fruits, 41-43, 123-25

g

Gallagher, Kim, 55
garlic, 175, 226-29, 237, 321
Gillman, Matthew, 41
ginger, 237
ginkgo biloba, 237-38
ginseng, 229-33, 253-54
Giovannucci, Edward, 69
glucose, 216, 298
glycogen, 146, 147-48, 184, 234
goiter, 260-62
Grinkov, Sergei, 55
Gullikson, Tim, 55

h

Halliwell, Barry, 43
hawthorne, 238
headaches, 233-34
  caffeine and, 132, 233
  chili peppers and, 158
  feverfew and, 236
  magnesium and, 281
  wine and, 336-37
healing, 200, 338-41
  ethinacea, 236
  ginseng and, 230
  pantothenic acid and, 307
  vitamin C and, 128
heart attacks
  aspirin and, 99, 101, 102
  folic acid and, 13, 17
  vitamin E and, 43-44
heart disease
  alcohol and, 73-74, 335-36
  aspirin and, 99, 101, 102
  beta-carotene and, 45-46, 66
  bioflavonoids and, 124
  caffeine and, 133
  coenzyme Q10 and, 169, 170-71, 172
  cruciferous vegetables and, 189, 190
  estrogen and, 245-50
  exercise and, 54-55
  folic acid and, 16-17, 25
  hawthorne and, 238
  iron and, 263, 265-66
  low-fat diet and, 216-17
  meat and, 283-85

Mediterranean diet and, 285-88
  obesity and, 297
  selenium and, 320, 321
  soy products and, 324, 328, 329
  vitamin B$_1$ and, 108-9
  vitamin C and, 128-29
  vitamin E and, 44
hemochromatosis, 263
hemoglobin, 96
hemorrhaging, 267, 268
Hennekens, Charles, 47
herbs
  harmful, 239-41
  helpful, 235-39, 241-42
hesperidin, 123-26
high blood pressure. See hypertension
HIV infections, 125
HMB (beta-hydroxy-beta-methylbutyrate), 88-89, 311-12
homocysteines
  balance of, 26-27
  dangers of, 24-25, 27-31
  folic acid and, 10, 13-14, 16-17, 32-36
  measuring, 31-32
Hopkins, Paul, 31
hormones
  DHEA, 201-3
  growth, 87-88
  nutritional therapy, 250-55
  replacement therapy, 245-50, 303-4
hypertension, 242-45
  caffeine and, 132, 133-34, 243
  calcium and, 138
  coenzyme Q10 and, 169, 170
  garlic and, 226, 229
  hawthorne and, 238
  homocysteines and, 24
  licorice and, 271-73
  magnesium and, 280
  obesity and, 295, 297-99
  pregnancy and, 136, 138, 139
  vitamin C and, 128
  vitamin D and, 194, 195-96

i

immune system, 255-58
  colds and, 174
  DHEA and, 201-2

Improve your health with other great books from Dr. Kenneth H. Cooper . . .

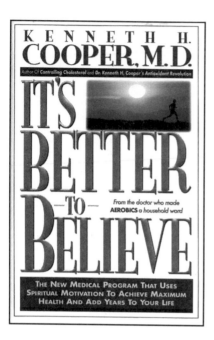

It's Better To Believe

The world's leading fitness expert shows readers the importance of being not just physically fit but spiritually fit as well. This comprehensive program uses spiritual resources to achieve maximum health, fitness, and longevity.

0-7852-8314-5 • Paperback • 256 pages

Dr. Kenneth H. Cooper's Antioxidant Revolution

The bestselling author who helped start the fitness boom offers a powerful program for improved health and well-being. Includes late-breaking research on antioxidants and how they can delay the signs of aging and prevent disease.

0-7852-7525-8 • Paperback • 240 pages

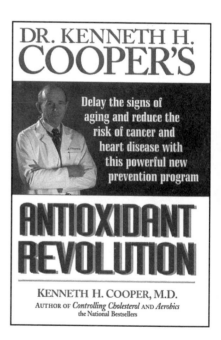